KV-411-506

PRIMARY FRCS
REVISION BOOK
MULTIPLE CHOICE QUESTIONS

Trust Library and Knowledge Services
Clinical Skills Centre
Queen Elizabeth Hospital
Telephone: 0191 4452935
Email: ghnt.medical.library@nhs.net

PRIMARY FRCS REVISION BOOK
MULTIPLE CHOICE QUESTIONS

Edited by:
MARY L. FORSLING, BSc, PhD
PETER H. ABRAHAMS, MB, BS
TIMOTHY J. CHAMBERS, MB, BS, BSc, PhD, MRCPath

PASTEST SERVICE
Hemel Hempstead
Hertfordshire
England

© 1982 PASTEST SERVICE
304 Galley Hill,
Hemel Hempstead, Herts. HP1 3LE
England. Tel. (0442) 52113-55550.

All rights reserved. No part of this publication may be reproduced, stored in a retrieval system, or transmitted, in any form or by any means, electronic, mechanical, photocopying, recording or otherwise without the prior permission of the copyright owner.
First published 1982
Reprinted 1986
ISBN 0-906896-07-X

British Library Cataloguing in Publication Data

Forsling, Mary L.
Primary FRCS revision book.
1. Surgery—Problems, exercises, etc.
I. Title II. Abrahams, Peter H.
III. Chambers, Timothy J.
617'.0076   R37.2
ISBN 0-906896-07-X

Phototypeset and Printed by Martin's of Berwick.

CONTENTS

Brackets indicate the number of questions in each subject

PREFACE

Comprehensive courses are arranged for undergraduate medical students so that any given subject is covered at the appropriate level. Equally, exposure to examinations during the course means that the student is aware of the standard required and is well prepared to take the University or College examinations at the end of the course. This is not the case at postgraduate level, so it is advisable to obtain some practice in answering question papers. The following text has been designed to fulfil this purpose.

The multiple choice question (MCQ) examination is part of the primary examination offered by the Royal College of Surgeons of the British Isles and Australasia. The ability to answer this paper satisfactorily is important as up to 20% of candidates may be eliminated and never given a *viva voce* examination as a result of poor performance in this section. In order to succeed in an MCQ test it is important to understand *why* a given answer is right and not merely to learn the right answer. If each section of this book is followed carefully, any gaps in the candidates knowledge should become apparent and furthermore they should gain extra confidence in sitting the examination.

M.F.

INTRODUCTION

This book contains 300 multiple choice questions. Initially there are 240 questions under the headings of anatomy, physiology and pathology. The last 60 questions are in the form of a complete practice examination also containing questions on each of these three topics, as found in the primary examination in surgery. Each question has a stem followed by five items which may be either true of false. Any combination of true or false is possible ranging from all true to all false. The correct answer code is given to every question together with an explanation. For convenience, questions are printed on the right hand side of the page with the answers and explanations on the following page. This format is followed throughout, except for the 60 questions which form the practice exam where the answers and explanations are given at the end. The explanation for each question is necessarily brief; if you are well-informed you should find your memory adequately refreshed. For a more detailed explanation the candidate should consult one of the texts given in the reading list. Attempt to answer each question in full before consulting the answer code. Each item may be marked true or false or a grid may be prepared (see below) so that you can enter in the answer as you proceed through the paper. Award yourself +1 for a correct response −1 for an incorrect one.

	A	B	C	D	E
23					
24					

To obtain the best value from the practice exam try to perform it under conditions as close as possible to those found in the examination. You should therefore try to select a time when you can be undisturbed for 2½ hours, the duration of the actual exam. Since there are 60 questions to be completed in this time, 2½ minutes should be allowed per question. It is important not to take longer than this otherwise you will not complete the paper satisfactorily. In the primary exam itself once you have decided whether a given response is true or false you have to mark your decision on an answer card. A marked card indicates "true", leaving it blank indicates "false", there is no opportunity to indicate "don't know". A blank card is taken to indicate that the response is false. The answer cards for the official exam will be read by a computer so it is essential that they are carefully completed in accordance with the instructions. The results of the practice exam may be scored using the answer codes at the end of this section; a score of 50% or more may be considered satisfactory. Let us hope you can do as well as this on the day.

SUGGESTED READING AND REFERENCE BOOKS

Anderson, J. R. *MUIRS TEXTBOOK OF PATHOLOGY* 5th edition 1979 pub. Churchill Livingstone.

Basmajian, J. V. *GRANT'S METHOD OF ANATOMY* 10th edition pub. Williams and Williams

Bell, G. H. Emslie-Smith D. & Paterson C. R. *TEXTBOOK OF PHYSIOLOGY AND BIOCHEMISTRY* pub. Churchill Livingstone 1980.

Ganong, W. F. *REVIEW OF MEDICAL PHYSIOLOGY* 9th edition pub. Lange Medical Publications, 1979.

Gillies, R. R. *LECTURE NOTES IN MEDICAL MICROBIOLOGY* 2nd edition pub. Blackwell 1978.

Goodman, L. S. & Gilman, A. *THE PHARMACOLOGICAL BASIS OF THERAPEUTICS* 6th edition pub. MacMillan 1980.

Gray, C. H. & Howarth P. J. N. *CLINICAL CHEMICAL PATHOLOGY* 9th edition pub. Edward Arnold 1979.

Hughes Jones, N. C. *LECTURE NOTES IN HAEMATOLOGY* 3rd edition pub. Blackwell 1979.

Kelman, G. R. *PHYSIOLOGY: A CLINICAL APPROACH* 3rd edition pub. Churchill Livingstone 1980.

McMinn, R. M. H. & Hutchings R. T. *COLOUR ATLAS OF ANATOMY* pub. Wolfe, Medical Publishers 1978.

Moore, K. L. *CLINICALLY ORIENTED ANATOMY* pub. Williams Wilkins 1980.

Mountcastle, V. B. *MEDICAL PHYSIOLOGY* 14th edition pub. Mosby 1980

Walter, O. B. & Israel M. S. *GENERAL PATHOLOGY* 5th edition pub. Churchill Livingstone 1979.

ANATOMY

HEAD AND NECK

1. The scalenus anterior muscle

    A is used as an accessory muscle of respiration
    B separates the subclavian artery and vein from the brachial plexus
    C is pierced by the phrenic nerve
    D is inserted into the first and second ribs
    E is anterior to the suprascapular artery

2. The parathyroid glands

    A develop from the third and fourth pharyngeal pouches
    B are supplied by branches of the external carotid and subclavian arteries
    C may sometimes be found in the posterior mediastinum
    D are exocrine glands
    E are closely related to the trachea

3. The pterygopalatine fossa

    A is bounded anteriorly by the sphenoid bone
    B transmits the maxillary nerve and artery
    C contains the posterior superior alveolar nerves
    D contains the greater (superficial) petrosal nerve
    E contains secretomotor fibres destined for the lacrimal gland

4. The inferior thyroid artery

    A branches after entering the thyroid gland
    B is closely related to the recurrent laryngeal nerve
    C gives off an oesophageal branch
    D is an anterior relation of the vagus nerve
    E arises from the common carotid artery

Answers overleaf

1. **A**

   The scalenus anterior muscle inserts into the scalene tubercle on the first rib, upper border. This muscle separates the subclavian vein anteriorly from the subclavian artery and brachial plexus which lie posterior to the muscle. The phrenic nerve lies on its anterior surface passing obliquely from lateral to medial and this nerve is pinned down on the muscle by the transverse cervical and suprascapular arteries. Lying just anterior to the arteries on the left-hand side is the terminal portion of the thoracic duct.

2. **A B E**

   These small endocrine glands, normally four in number, lie in the posterior part of the thyroid gland receiving their blood supply from the superior thyroid (ext. carotid) and inferior thyroid (subclavian) arteries. As they develop with the thymus gland, it is not uncommon to find parathyroid ectopic tissue in the superior mediastinum, but not in the posterior mediastinum.

3. **B C E**

   This fossa, also known as the sphenopalatine fossa, has as its posterior border the sphenoid bone. The fossa's contents include the maxillary nerve (V^2), pterygopalatine ganglion, and the third part of the maxillary artery with accompanying veins. The pterygopalatine ganglion is the relay station for parasympathetic fibres which, after synapsing, continue via the zygomatic and lacrimal nerves to the lacrimal gland. The greater petrosal nerve joins the deep petrosal nerve to form the nerve of the pterygoid canal (vidian nerve), and it is this nerve that carries the preganglionic fibres into the fossa and towards the ganglion.

4. **B C**

   The inferior thyroid artery is a branch off the thyrocervical trunk which arises from the first part of the subclavian artery. It branches outside the pretracheal fascia. The vagus nerve lies anterior to the inferior thyroid artery, but its branch, the recurrent laryngeal nerve, is often entwined with various branches of the artery. It is quite easy to damage the nerve if one is not careful when ligating the inferior thyroid artery during thyroidectomy.

5. **The lingual nerve**

   A supplies the mucous membrane of the anterior two-thirds of the tongue
   B passes under the submandibular duct
   C is a branch of the anterior division of the mandibular nerve
   D carries parasympathetic fibres to the submandibular ganglion
   E passes into a canal within the mandible itself

6. **The parotid gland**

   A is a serous gland
   B is in direct contact with the internal carotid artery
   C has a glenoid lobe which lies behind the mandibular joint, in close contact with the external acoustic meatus
   D encloses the "pes anserinus"
   E lies within the parotid fascia which is an extension of the investing layer of the deep cervical fascia

7. **The temporomandibular joint**

   A has bony surfaces covered with hyaline cartilage
   B is commonly dislocated in a forwards direction
   C contains a fibrous disc which is pulled forward by the lateral pterygoid muscle
   D is more stable when the teeth are occluded
   E is protracted by the medial pterygoid muscles and the anterior belly of digastric

8. **The costocervical trunk**

   A arises from the third part of the subclavian artery
   B arises anterior to scalenus anterior muscle
   C gives off the transverse cervical artery
   D gives off the superior intercostal artery
   E passes anterior to the phrenic nerve

Answers overleaf

5. A B D

The lingual nerve is a branch of the posterior division of the mandibular nerve which carries preganglionic secretomotor fibres which supply the submandibular and sublingual glands. The other major branch of the posterior division is the inferior alveolar (dental) nerve, which enters the mandible at the lingular and passes along its own bony canal within the mandible. The lingual nerve lies just alongside the internal border of the mandible above the mylohyoid line.

6. A C D E

The parotid gland is in contact with the retromandibular vein and external carotid artery, but separated from the internal carotid artery by the posterior belly of digastric, stylohyoid muscle and styloid process. The "pes anserinus" or goose's foot the 5 branches of the facial nerve which emerge from within the gland itself. The fact that the gland is enclosed within an envelope of the investing cervical fascia explains why mumps is so painful due to stretching of this fascia.

7. B C D

The bony surfaces of the temporomandibular joint are covered with fibrocartilage. There is no hyaline cartilage in this joint. The muscle of protraction is the lateral pterygoid which is also most important in aiding gravity in opening the mouth. The digastric muscle is also involved in opening, but the medial pterygoid muscles close the jaw and, in co-operation with the lateral pterygoids, control sideways grinding movements.

8. D

The costocervical trunk arises from the second part of the subclavian artery which lies posterior to the scalenus anterior muscle. The phrenic nerve lies on the anterior surface of the muscle where it is pinned down by the transverse cervical and suprascapular arteries, both of which are branches of the thyrocervical trunk. The costocervical gives rise to the superior intercostal artery supplying the upper two intercostal spaces and a branch to the deep cervical musculature.

9. **In the tongue**

    A the vallate papillae are supplied by the glossopharyngeal nerve

    B lymph from the posterior third of the tongue drains bilaterally into the jugulo-omohyoid nodes

    C the palatoglossus muscle is supplied by the hypoglossal nerve

    D the intrinsic muscles are derived from suboccipital myotomes

    E the styloglossus muscle is supplied by the glossopharyngeal nerve

10. **The thyroid gland**

    A only receives its blood supply from the external carotid and subclavian arteries

    B in its resting state is composed of distended vesicles containing colloid

    C develops from the foramen caecum situated at the junction of the anterior third and posterior two thirds of the tongue

    D may include an upward projection generally situated on the left

    E may be found in a suprahyoid position

11. **The vertebral artery**

    A arises from the second part of the subclavian artery posterior to scalenus anterior muscle

    B lies anterior to the inferior thyroid artery

    C passes through the C7 foramen transversarium

    D meets its opposite artery to form the basilar artery within the cranium

    E lies anterior to the lateral mass of the atlas

12. **The mandibular branch of the trigeminal nerve supplies the**

    A tensor palati muscle

    B mylohyoid muscle

    C posterior belly of digastric

    D mastoid antrum and air cells

    E tensor tympani muscle

Answers overleaf

9. A B D

All the intrinsic muscles of the tongue are supplied by the hypoglossal nerve, as are the extrinsic muscles with the single exception of the palatoglossus muscle which is supplied through the pharyngeal plexus. The styloglossus is therefore supplied by the hypoglossal nerve which must not be confused with the stylopharyngeus muscle, which is the only muscle supplied directly by the glossopharyngeal nerve.

10. B D

The major blood supply to the gland is from the external carotid and subclavian arteries, but there is also sometimes a thyroidea ima artery. The origin of the gland is from the foramen caecum which is situated at the junction of the anterior two thirds and posterior third of the tongue. The left lobular projection is the pyramidal lobe. The gland itself is not found inferior to the thyroid cartilage, but aberrant thyroid tissue is often found along the developmental tract. This may lead to thyroglossal cysts lying in both the suprahyoid and infrahyoid positions.

11. D

The vertebral artery is a direct branch of the first part of the subclavian artery and lies posterior to the tortuous inferior thyroid artery. Normally, it passes through the C6 foramen transversarium though the vertebral veins often do pass through the C7 foramina. After passing superiorly through each foramen, it passes posterior to the lateral mass of the atlas; enters the foramen magnum and, joining its opposite number, becomes the basilar artery lying on the clivus.

12. A B E

A branch of the mandibular nerve to the medial pterygoid muscle also supplies both the tensor palati and tensor tympani muscles. The inferior alveolar (dental) nerve gives a small twig to the mylohyoid muscle which also supplies the anterior belly of digastric. The posterior belly of the digastric muscle is supplied by the facial (VII) nerve.

Upper Limb

13. **The radial nerve**

    A   is the main branch of the posterior cord of the brachial
        plexus
    B   is usually derived from the posterior primary rami of
        C5, 6, 7, 8 and the T1 nerve roots
    C   is the main nerve supply to the extensor compartments
        of the arm and forearm
    D   gives rise to the anterior interosseous nerve
    E   supplies the extensor aspect of the radial three and a half
        digits

14. **The carpal tunnel syndrome (compression of the median nerve
    by the flexor retinaculum) will usually cause**

    A   wasting of adductor pollicis
    B   wasting of opponens pollicis
    C   wasting of flexor pollicis longus
    D   sensory loss over the skin of the ring finger
    E   sensory loss over the thenar eminence

15. **The following muscles contribute to the extensor expansion of
    the fingers:**

    A   extensor digitorum longus
    B   extensor indicis
    C   palmar interossei
    D   extensor pollicis longus
    E   the two medial lumbricals

16. **Branches of the posterior cord of the brachial plexus are the**

    A   axillary nerve
    B   lateral pectoral nerve
    C   long thoracic nerve
    D   nerve to rhomboids
    E   nerve to teres major

Answers overleaf

13. A C E

The other branches off the posterior cord are the axillary thoracodorsal, and upper and lower subscapular nerves. All the brachial plexus roots of origin are from anterior primary rami. The radial nerve passes through supinator muscle in the forearm and gives rise to the posterior interosseous nerve; it is the median nerve which has the anterior interosseous branch.

14. B D

The adductor pollicis is the odd one out with regards to the small muscles of the thumb. It is normally ulnar innervated whilst the others are median nerve innervated, such as opponens pollicis. The flexor pollicis longus however, will be unaffected by wrist compression as it is innervated by the anterior interosseous nerve in the forearm. The skin of the medial part of the ring finger will be affected by the compression, but the thenar skin is supplied by the palmar branch of the median nerve, which passes superficial to the flexor retinaculum and is therefore unaffected in this patient.

15. A B C E

The dorsal extensor expansion of the fingers has contribution from the extensor digitorum longus, extensor indicis, both the dorsal and palmar interossei and the four lumbrical muscles which pass from the flexor digitorum longus into the dorsal hood and expansion. There is no extensor expansion of the thumb.

16. A E

The branches of the posterior cord are the radial, axillary, thoracodorsal (to latissimus dorsi), upper and lower subscapular nerves. The lateral pectoral nerve is a branch from the lateral cord to pectoralis major. The long thoracic nerve (Bell) to serratus anterior originates from the roots C5, C6 and C7 directly. The nerve to rhomboids (dorsal scapular) is also a branch from the C5 root directly.

17. **The median nerve**

    A arises from the medial and lateral divisions of the brachial plexus
    B at the cubital fossa passes between the two heads of pronator teres
    C at the wrist is situated between palmaris longus and flexor carpi radialis tendons
    D crosses centrally over the flexor retinaculum
    E if involved in the carpal tunnel syndrome may give rise to anaesthesia over the thenar eminence

18. **Structures which pass superficially to the flexor retinaculum are the**

    A ulnar nerve—palmar branch
    B palmar branch of median nerve
    C anterior interosseous nerve
    D the tendon of palmaris longus
    E flexor pollicis longus tendon

19. **The anterior interosseous nerve**

    A supplies pronator teres
    B supplies flexor pollicis longus
    C ends in the anterior part of the capsule of the wrist joint, which it supplies
    D supplies a small area of skin overlying the anterior surface of the wrist joint
    E supplies the medial two lumbrical muscles

20. **The axilla contains**

    A the trunks of the brachial plexus
    B superior thoracic artery
    C latissimus dorsi muscle in its medial wall
    D the dorsal scapular nerve
    E the long thoracic nerve in its medial wall

Answers overleaf

17. B C

The median nerve originates from the medial and lateral cords of the brachial plexus and at the wrist passes deep to the flexor retinaculum centrally. However, a small palmar branch passes superficial to the retinaculum and is therefore unaffected in carpal tunnel syndrome where the anaesthesia involving the digits does not affect the thenar eminence. A person not possessing a palmaris longus may find he has a palpable, tender median nerve just proximal to the wrist joint.

18. A B D

The ulnar nerve and artery as well as its palmar branch lie superficial to the flexor retinaculum. Though the median nerve passes deep to the retinaculum, its major branch in the forearm, the anterior interosseous nerve, lies very deep in the forearm flexor compartment and usually terminates in the forearm in pronator quadratus which it supplies. Another muscle this nerve supplies is the flexor pollicis longus which lies in its own compartment within the carpal tunnel deep to the flexor retinaculum.

19. B C

Pronator teres is supplied by the median nerve directly as it passes between the muscle's two heads. The anterior interosseous nerve has no cutaneous branches. The medial two lumbricals are supplied by the ulnar nerve whereas the lateral two lumbricals are supplied by the palmar digital branches of the median nerve.

20. B E

The axilla contains the brachial plexus, but it is the cords that lie here, whereas the trunks lie in the posterior triangle of the neck. The tendon of latissimus dorsi lies in the axilla and is one of its posterior borders. The dorsal scapular nerve is the nerve to the rhomboid muscles (C5) and lies superior and posterior to the axilla. The long thoracic nerve (Bell) lies along the medial border of serratus anterior to which it sends numerous twigs. This nerve must be treated with respect when removing axillary lymph nodes during a radical mastectomy!

21. In the shoulder joint

A flexion is produced by clavicular head of pectoralis major
B adduction is initiated by supraspinatus
C deltoid is the principal adductor
D extension is produced by latissimus dorsi and the long head of triceps
E lateral rotation is performed by subscapularis and teres major

22. At the elbow joint

A anconeus muscle is involved in flexion
B brachioradialis muscle lies just anterior to the joint before inserting into the coronoid process
C the common extensor origin of muscles lies medially
D the ulnar collateral ligament inserts into the anular ligament
E fat pads lie in the coronoid fossa, between the synovial membrane and the capsular ligament

THORAX

23. The coronary sinus

A originates from the sinus venosus
B receives venous blood from the anterior cardiac veins
C receives venous blood from the great and middle cardiac veins
D opens directly into the right atrium
E receives venous blood from the venae cordis minimae (Thebesian veins)

24. The aortic arch

A is developed from the third left pharyngeal arch artery
B is crossed anteriorly on the left by the vagus and phrenic nerves
C is in communication with the pulmonary vein in the fetus
D lies in both the superior and posterior mediastinum
E arches backwards over the left main bronchus

Answers overleaf

21. A D

Supraspinatus and deltoid are both abductors and although many books rate supraspinatus of prime importance in the initial stages of abduction, it is quite evident to the patient with a paralysed deltoid that early abduction is nearly impossible. A useful test is to watch the patient remove something from a trouser pocket. The lateral rotators are infraspinatus and teres minor; subscapularis and teres major are medial rotators.

22. E

This synovial hinge joint is between humerus and the upper ends of radius and ulna. The brachialis and brachioradialis muscles lie anterior to the joint, but it is the brachialis which inserts into the coronoid process of the ulna. The anconeus muscle is a small extensor muscle acting with triceps. The forearm flexors and pronator teres originate from the medial epicondyle, whereas the extensor origin is the lateral epicondyle. The triangular-shaped radial collateral ligament inserts into the anular ligament which stabilises the radial head, resisting dislocation. The ulnar collateral ligament has three bands which insert into the olecranon and coronoid processes.

23. A C D

The coronary sinus is about 4 cm long and lies in the atrioventricular groove posteriorly opening directly into the right atrium. Its tributaries include the great cardiac vein, the posterior vein of the left ventricle, the middle cardiac vein and the small cardiac vein. The oblique vein of the left atrium also drains into the sinus. The anterior cardiac veins and venae cordis minimal drain directly into the left atrium.

24. B E

The aortic arch develops from the fourth left pharyngeal arch, the third becomes the internal carotid. In the fetus, the arch and the pulmonary artery are in communication via the ductus arteriosus which normally shrivels into the fibrous ligamentum arteriosum of the adult. The arch of the aorta is by definition only in the superior mediastinum, as it is the descending aorta which lies in the posterior mediastinum, below T4 vertebral level.

25. The lymphatic drainage of the female breast

A of one side communicates with that of the other side
B is mainly to the lateral axillary lymph nodes of the same side
C is initially only to the sub-areolar plexus
D includes the lymph nodes along the internal thoracic artery of the same side
E follows the subscapular vessels to the posterior axillary lymph nodes

26. The thymus gland

A is the principal content of the anterior mediastinum
B is developed from the 4th pharyngeal pouch
C is larger in old age
D is made up of small round endodermal cells
E descends anterior to the brachiocephalic veins

27. Surface markings on chest examination include the

A third thoracic vertebra at the level of the tracheal bifurcation
B right nipple in a non-pendulous breast as the extreme limit of the right cupola of the diaphragm
C suprasternal notch as the level of the third thoracic vertebra
D aortic arch which lies at the level of the fourth thoracic vertebra
E xiphisternal joint at the level of the disc between ninth and tenth thoracic vertebrae

28. The sympathetic chain

A is formed from the peripheral processes of the connector cell bodies passing out in the anterior roots of T1-L2 inclusive
B carries parasympathetic fibres below L2
C lies anterior to the common iliac vessels
D lies anterior to the segmental vessels, i.e. lumbar arteries and veins
E lies posterior to the psoas fascia

Answers overleaf

25. D E

Initially, the lymphatic drainage is to both the subareolar plexus superficially and the submammary deep plexus. There is no direct communication between the lymphatics of one breast to the other, but pathology in one may metastasize to the other due to blocked lymphatic channels. The breast mainly drains to the axillary nodes (pectoral, posterior and central), the lateral axillary nodes being the major drainage site of the arm and not the breast.

26. A D E

The thymus develops ventrally from the third pharyngeal pouch with the inferior parathyroid glands which develop dorsally from the same pouch. The thymus is largest in childhood and regresses in old age. The small round endodermal cells are the thymocytes, the lamellated keratinous bodies are Hassall's corpuscles.

27. B D E

The classical level of both aortic arch and bifurcation of the trachea are the level of T4. In fact, during respiration, the bifurcation moves between T4 and T6. The suprasternal (jugular) notch is at the level of T2, whilst the manubriosternal joint is at the T4 level. The upper limit of the right cupola is also the upper level of the liver border.

28. A D

The sympathetic chain goes from the base of the skull to the coccyx, but never carries parasympathetic fibres. The iliac vessels are aortic branches, not segmental vessels. The chain lies behind the iliac vessels, but anterior to the segmental vessels such as the lumbar vessels. On passing inferiorly, the sympathetic chain lies on the psoas fascia between the psoas muscle and the vertebral column.

29. The clavicle

A   although a long bone, develops primarily in cartilage
B   is the last bone to ossify in the fetus
C   is one of the last bones to stop growing
D   has no secondary centre of ossification
E   provides attachments for the sternomastoid, deltoid
      and trapezius muscles

30. The diaphragm

A   is supplied by the phrenic and intercostal nerves
B   is developed from the septum-transversum and C4 myotome
C   has an opening in the central tendon which transmits the
      right phrenic nerve
D   has a right dome which is higher than the left dome
E   has a left crus which is larger than the right crus

31. The oesophagus

A   is 25 cm long
B   passes behind the left bronchus in the thorax
C   consists of only smooth muscle
D   is mainly lined by stratified squamous epithelium
E   drains all its blood into the azygos and hemiazygos systems

32. The trachea

A   has a total length of about 10 cm in the adult
B   is directly related to the right vagus nerve
C   is directly related to the left subclavian artery
D   is prevented from collapsing during inspiration by
      incomplete rings of elastic cartilage
E   is directly related to the arch of the azygos vein

Answers overleaf

29. C E

The clavicle is the first bone to ossify in the fetus and one of the last bones to stop growing in the adult. Most long bones ossify in cartilage. The clavicle, however, is an exception as it ossifies in membrane, and the medial end becomes fibrocartilagenous. A secondary centre of ossification appears here at about the 18th year, and joins the body of the clavicle at about 25.

30. A B C D

The sole motor supply of the diaphragm is the phrenic nerve, but the sensory supply is shared by the phrenic (majority) and the intercostals peripherally. The opening in the central tendon is for the inferior vena cava. The right dome or cupola is normally higher due to the underlying liver. The right crus is larger originating from L1, 2, 3 bodies, whereas the left crus only originates from L1 and L2. The right crus fibres cross over the midline to encircle the oesphagus and form part of its sphincter mechanism.

31. A B D

The muscular wall of the oesphagus consists of both smooth and striped muscle. The upper third is striped and the lower two thirds smooth, there being a mixture in some parts. The arterial supply to the oesphagus includes branches of the inferior thyroid, aorta and left gastric arteries. The venous blood drains into the inferior thyroid, azygos and left gastric veins. The communications between azygos and left gastric veins are a clinically important site of portosystemic venous anastomosis.

32. B C E

The total length of the trachea is about 15 cm., and its shape is maintained by the horseshoe-like rings of hyaline cartilage. There are normally 15-20 of these rings ending in the bikini-shaped inferior carinal cartilage. The arch of the azygos vein lies between the lung and pleural sac laterally and the oesphagus and trachea medially.

ABDOMEN

33. The right hepatic artery

A   usually gives off the cystic artery
B   usually passes posterior to the common hepatic duct
C   usually lies anterior to the portal vein
D   supplies the caudate lobe of the liver
E   supplies a Riedel's lobe when present

34. The porta hepatis

A   is enclosed by the free edge of the lesser omentum
B   contains the hepatic veins
C   contains the portal vein overlying the hepatic artery
D   contains the entire length of the cystic duct
E   contains lymph nodes which drain from the gall bladder

35. The spermatic cord contains the

A   ilioinguinal nerve
B   vas deferens
C   lymph nodes from the testes
D   sympathetic nerve fibres
E   branches of the inferior epigastric artery

36. Para-umbilical pain could be due to pathology in the

A   periphery of the diaphragm
B   vermiform appendix
C   right kidney
D   dermatome of the 8th thoracic spinal nerve
E   skin of the scrotum

Answers overleaf

33. A B C E

Although the relations of the hepatic artery to the cystic artery, common hepatic duct and portal vein are as described, it is very important for the surgeon to remember that there are numerous anomalies in this region. Beware! The caudate and quadrate lobes of the liver are functionally part of the left lobe, and supplied by the left hepatic artery.

34. A E

The hepatic veins pass from the liver's posterior surface to drain into the inferior vena cava. The portal vein lies deep to the hepatic artery and common bile duct, but only the distal end of the cystic duct is in the porta hepatis.

35. B D E

The ilioinguinal nerve (L1) runs outside the cord, whilst the only lymphatics within the cord are the channels, no nodes are reached until the pelvis (iliac nodes). The major branch of importance from the inferior epigastric artery is the cremasteric artery to the cremaster muscle of the spermatic cord.

36. A B C

The para-umbilical region is supplied by the T10 spinal nerve and it is through the mechanism of referred pain that pain from the appendix, small bowel, testes and kidney is felt in this region. Remember also that the diaphragm's sensory supply is from the lower five intercostal nerves. The scrotal skin, however, is innervated by the 1st lumbar spinal nerve, although its contents, the testes, are from T10.

37. **The common bile duct**

   A lies in the free edge of the greater omentum
   B is anterior to the portal vein and to the left of the
      hepatic artery
   C is in a groove on the posterior aspect of the pancreas in
      front of the right renal vein
   D may open into the duodenum independent of the
      pancreatic duct
   E is anterior to the first part of the duodenum

38. **The duodenum**

   A is approximately 25 cm long
   B has the origin of the inferior mesenteric artery crossing
      its third part
   C at its junction with the jejunum is fixed to the left psoas
      muscle by a suspensory ligamentous structure
   D in its second part is related to the hilum of the
      right kidney
   E in its first part is related anteriorly to the inferior surface
      of the right lobe of the liver

39. **The ligamentum teres of the liver**

   A is the obliterated left umbilical vein
   B is contained in the free edge of the coronary
      ligament
   C is continuous with the median umbilical ligament
   D passes over the superior border of the liver
   E is continuous with the ligamentum venosum

40. **The inferior vena cava**

   A passes through the diaphragm at the level of the
      8th thoracic vertebra
   B runs in a deep groove on the posterior aspect of the liver
   C is related to the fourth part of the duodenum
   D lies to the left of the aorta as it ascends in the abdomen
   E is formed by the union of the common iliac veins in front
      of the right common iliac artery

Answers overleaf

37. **C D**

The common bile duct lies in the free edge of the *lesser* omentum and to the right of the hepatic artery. It passes inferiorly from the lesser omental free edge posterior to the first part of the duodenum to open into the descending (second) part of the duodenum.

38. **A D E**

The origin of the superior mesenteric artery crosses over the third part of the duodenum; the inferior mesenteric artery is only related to the lower border of the third part. The so-called 'suspensory ligament' is, in fact, smooth muscle fibres which may blend with psoas fascia.

39. **A E**

The ligamentum teres is contained in the free edge of the falciform ligament. It is not continuous with the median umbilical ligament which is the remnant of the urachus from the bladder. The ligamentum teres lies in a deep groove on the visceral inferior surface of the liver and is functionally continuous in the fetus with the ductus venosus (ligamentum venosum of the adult).

40. **A B**

The inferior vena cava is related to the third part of the duodenum and lies to the right hand side of the aorta as it ascends the abdomen. It is indeed formed by the union of the two common iliac veins, but these lie behind the right common iliac artery.

41. The pancreas

    A   is an anterior relation of the left kidney
    B   derives its blood supply from the splenic artery
    C   extends into both supracolic and infracolic compartments
    D   is pierced by the middle colic artery
    E   lies posterior to the portal vein

42. The following structures pass beneath the inguinal ligament:

    A   psoas major muscle
    B   femoral branch of genitofemoral nerve
    C   long saphenous vein
    D   superficial epigastric vein
    E   external pudendal vein

PELVIS

43. The deep perineal pouch contains the

    A   deep dorsal vein of the penis
    B   sphincter urethrae muscle ('External sphincter')
    C   bulb of penile urethra
    D   deep transverse perineal muscle
    E   greater vestibular glands (Bartholin)

44. The ureter

    A   contains circular and longitudinal smooth muscle arranged
        in spirals
    B   is lined with columnar epithelium
    C   receives its nerve supply from L2, L3 and L4
    D   develops from the mesonephric duct
    E   radiologically lies on the tips of the transverse processes
        of the lumbar vertebrae

Answers overleaf

41. A B C

The tail of the pancreas crosses the left kidney on its way towards the hilum of the spleen. Most of the gland lies in the supracolic compartment, but a small portion along its inferior border lies within the infracolic compartment. The middle colic artery arises from its lower border, it is the superior mesenteric trunk itself that pierces the gland. The formation of the portal vein from splenic and mesenteric veins lies behind the neck of the pancreas.

42. B

The psoas major muscle does not pass beneath the inguinal ligament; it is the tendon that lies deep to the femoral artery beneath the ligament. The long saphenous vein terminates distal to the ligament some 3-4 cm lateral and inferior to the pubic tubercle, passing through the cribriform fascia to join the femoral vein. The superficial epigastric vein crosses above the ligament whilst another tributary of the long saphenous, the external pudendal vein, does not cross the ligament at all.

43. A B D

The membranous urethra, surrounding sphincter urethrae muscle and the bulbourethral glands (Cowper) are all within the deep pouch, i.e. deep to the perineal membrane and superficial to the superior fascia of the urogenital diaphragm. The penile bulb of course sits on the perineal membrane and with the greater vestibular glands both lie in the superficial pouch or space.

44. A D E

The ureter and bladder are lined with transitional epithelium whereas the vas deferens is lined with columnar epithelium. The sympathetic nerve supply to the ureter is from the L1 and L2 vertebral levels. Remember that there is no sympathetic outflow below L2!

45. The prostate gland

A is separated from the rectal fascia by the prostatic fascia of Denonvilliers
B lies against the inferior fascia of the urogenital diaphragm
C has a prostatic plexus of veins into which drains the deep dorsal vein of the penis
D is traversed by the vasa deferentia
E is supplied by the inferior vesical arteries

46. The rectum

A has a very short mesentery
B is supplied mainly by the superior mesenteric artery
C is a site of portosystemic venous anastomosis
D normally has three taeniae coli
E has anteroposterior and lateral curves

47. The following structures lie between the ureter and the peritoneum in the pelvis:

A Vas deferens (in the male)
B obturator nerve
C uterine artery (in the female)
D superior vesical artery
E sympathetic chain or trunk

48. Contents of the superficial perineal pouch include the

A perineal body
B membranous urethra
C bulbospongiosus muscle
D bulbourethral glands of Cowper
E perineal nerve

Answers overleaf

Anatomy

45. A C E

The prostate gland lies on the levatores ani and its apex abuts against the superior fascia of the urogenital diaphragm. The inferior fascia is better known as the perineal membrane. The gland itself is transversed by the ejactulatory ducts which are formed by the union of the vasa deferentia and seminal vesicles, both of which lie posterior to the gland. These ducts open beside the prostatic utricle into the prostatic urethra.

46. C E

The rectum has no mesentry, its upper third being covered by peritoneum on the anterior and lateral surfaces, the middle third is covered only anteriorly, and the lower part of the rectum is surrounded by the pelvic fascia. Its arterial supply is from the superior rectal (haemorrhoidal) branch of the inferior mesenteric artery. The rectum, like the appendix, has no taeniae coli, but a continuous tube of longitudinal muscle fibres.

47. A C

The vas deferens in the male and uterine artery in the female are the only structures to pass between the ureter and pelvic peritoneum. The obturator nerve lies lateral to the ureter along the lateral pelvic wall. The superior vesical artery is a visceral branch of the internal iliac artery and runs posterior to the ureter, often supplying it inferiorly. The sacral sympathetic trunks lie behind the iliac vessels on the posterolateral walls of the pelvis.

48. C E

The superficial perineal pouch or space is limited by the perineal membrane which lies deep and the limitations of the urogenital triangle anteroposteriorly. Therefore, the perineal body or central tendon of the perineum lies posterior to the diaphragm and the membranous urethra lies deep to the perineal membrance in the deep perineal pouch. Here the membranous urethra is surrounded by the sphincter urethrae muscle in which are embedded the bulbourethral glands of Cowper. Their ducts pierce the perineal membrane to drain into the bulbous urethra.

49. The uterus

A has a serous coat on all surfaces
B is supplied by branches of the external iliac artery
C is drained by lymphatics to the superficial inguinal nodes
D receives a sensory nerve supply by way of the hypogastric plexi
E normally lies in a position of retroversion and anteflexion.

50. The superficial inguinal lymph node drainage area includes the

A skin of the superior part of the buttock
B lower vagina and labia
C upper portion of the uterine body
D the anus above the pectinate line
E the little toe nail

51. The lesser sciatic foramen transmits the

A posterior femoral cutaneous nerve of thigh
B nerve to obturator internus
C nerve to quadratus femoris
D inferior gluteal artery
E pudendal nerve and artery

52. The bladder

A is composed solely of smooth muscle lined by a distensible mucous membrane
B is separated from the pubic symphysis by areolar tissue
C may receive part of its blood supply from the inferior epigastric artery
D may be attached to the umbilicus by the medial umbilical ligament
E develops from both endodermal and mesodermal origins

Answers overleaf

49. C D

Posteriorly, the pelvic peritoneum is very adherent, but it is reflected off the uterus to form the broad ligament laterally and at the base of the bladder anteriorly. The uterine blood supply is from branches of the internal iliac vessesls. Though most of the lymphatics of the uterus drain to the internal iliac group of nodes, a small area at the fundus drains via the round ligament to the superficial inguinal nodes. About 80% of women have an anteverted anteflexed uterus, in retroversion the uterine fundus is directed backwards—this is a physical sign, not a disease!

50. A B C E

The superficial inguinal lymph nodes receive nearly all the lymph vessels from the skin of the lower limbs, perineum and buttocks. These nodes also drain the anus below the pectinate line, lower vagina, labia and a small region of the uterus which drains via the round ligament of the uterus to the groin. The upper portion of the anus drains via the inferior mesenteric vessels to mesenteric nodes and eventually to the aortic nodes.

51. B E

The posterior femoral cutaneous nerve of the thigh often runs superficially with the sciatic nerve exiting the greater sciatic foramen inferior to the piriformis muscle. The small nerve to quadratus femoris and the inferior gluteal nerve also both exit the gluteal region through the greater sciatic foramen usually below piriformis and just superior to the ischial spine. The lesser sciatic foramen transmits the pudendal vessels and nerve, the obturator internus muscle and its nerve and the two gamelli muscles.

52. A B C E

The medial umbilical ligaments are the folds of peritoneum which cover the remnants of the umbilical arteries. The median umbilical ligament is the remains of the urachus which attaches the bladder to the umbilicus. Occasionally, a patent urachus may allow urine to be voided via the umbilicus—an interesting proof of this connection.

LOWER LIMB

53. **The popliteus**

A arises from the popliteal surface of the tibia below the soleal line
B is supplied by a branch of the tibial nerve
C pulls the medial meniscus posteriorly
D is a medial rotator of the femur on the tibia
E lies outside the capsule of the knee joint

54. **The flexor hallucis longus**

A is a multipennate muscle whose fibres arise from the flexor surface of fibula
B is very important for maintaining the medial longitudinal arch of the foot
C tendon grooves the posterior process of the calcaneum
D tendon is inserted into the base of the proximal phalanx of the big toe
E is supplied by the tibial nerve

55. **The femoral nerve supplies**

A gluteus minimus muscle
B rectus femoris muscle
C the skin over the lateral malleolus
D iliacus muscle
E the ankle joint

56. **The branches of the lumbar plexus are the**

A nerve to piriformis
B iliohypogastric nerve
C nerve to psoas major
D pudendal nerve
E genitofemoral nerve

Answers overleaf

53. B

The popliteus muscle arises above the soleal line on the tibia. It is the muscle which 'unlocks' the fully extended knee prior to flexion and rotates laterally the femur on the tibia and pulls the lateral meniscus posteriorly. It lies within the capsule of the knee joint and its tendon may therefore be visualised in a knee arthrogram X-ray.

54. A B E

The flexor hallucis longus is rather special in man as it originates on the lateral side (fibula) of the lower leg and yet inserts into the hallux which is medial. Its tendon grooves the posterior process of the talus not the calcaneum. The tendon does insert into the big toe, but into the distal phalanx where it gets the maximum mechanical advantage. All the muscles of the posterior flexor compartment that act upon the foot are supplied by the tibial branch of the sciatic nerve.

55. B D

The gluteus minimus muscle is supplied by the superior gluteal nerve. The femoral nerve supplies the skin over the lower medial part of the leg and medial malleolus via its saphenous branch (L4). The femoral nerve also supplies the hip and knee joints, but the ankle joint is supplied by the tibial and deep peroneal nerves.

56. B C E

The lumbar plexus is formed from the anterior (ventral) rami of the first four lumbar spinal nerves. It is formed within the psoas muscle, and most of its nerves exit the psoas along its lateral border although the obturator nerve lies medial and the genitofemoral nerve often pierces the psoas anteriorly. The nerve to piriformis is a direct branch from the sacral plexus and the pudendal nerve from S2, 3 and 4.

57. The hip joint

A   is supplied by the nerve to rectus femoris
B   is supplied by the nerve to quadratus femoris
C   is supplied by the obturator nerve
D   has a posterior capsule attached to the greater
     trochanter
E   is supported most strongly by the ischiofemoral ligament

58. A lesion of the common peroneal nerve may

A   be produced by a fracture of the neck of the fibula
B   abolish active extension of the hallux
C   cause foot drop
D   abolish inversion of the foot
E   produce anaesthesia of the sole of the foot

59. The knee joint

A   is essentially a modified hinge joint with the ability to
     rotate when extended
B   is reinforced by ligaments, the strongest of which is the tibial
     collateral ligament
C   contains cruciate ligaments which lie within the
     synovial membrane
D   receives its nerve supply from only the femoral and
     sciatic nerves
E   has a lateral meniscus, to which popliteus is attached
     posteriorly

60. The sciatic nerve

A   divides into tibial and common peroneal nerves at a variable
     level in the lower limb
B   lies under cover of gluteus maximus midway between the
     greater trochanter and the ischial tuberosity
C   is derived from the anterior rami of the L4, 5 and S1, 2
     and 3 nerves
D   supplies the gluteal muscles
E   is the main nerve supplying the adductor magnus

Answers overleaf

57. A B C

Hilton's law states that a joint receives its nerve supply from the same nerves that innervate the muscles acting across that joint. Hence the hip joint is innervated by numerous nerves including the femoral, obturator, sciatic and nerve to quadratus femoris. The capsule of the hip joint anteriorly is attached to the trochanters, but posteriorly only attaches as far as half way down the femoral neck. Though strong the ischiofemoral ligament is not so strong as the inverted "Y"-shaped iliofemoral ligament of Bigelow. This latter ligament passes from the anterior inferior iliac spine to each end of the intertrochanteric line.

58. A B C

The common peroneal branch of the sciatic nerve winds around the neck of the fibula prior to dividing into the superficial and deep peroneal nerves. These latter nerves control eversion and dorsiflexion which, if lost, give rise to an inverted plantarflexed foot, i.e. foot drop. Inversion would not be completely lost as tibialis posterior is innervated by the tibial nerve and it is this muscle in combination with tibialis anterior that produces inversion. The sole of the foot is innervated by the medial and lateral plantar branches of the tibial nerve.

59. B E

The knee joint has the ability to rotate, but only when flexed—try it on yourself. Its nerve supply follows Hilton's law and is therefore supplied by not only the femoral and sciatic nerve, but also a twig from the obturator nerve. The cruciate ligaments, which resist the anteroposterior movements of the femur on the tibia, are both intracapsular, but extrasynovial, due to the development of the synovial compartments of the knee joint.

60. A B C

The sciatic nerve is the largest in the body and is derived from the lumbosacral plexus (L4, 5; S1, 2 and 3). The gluteus maximus is supplied by the inferior gluteal nerve whilst the gluteus medius and minimus are supplied by the superior gluteal nerve. Although supplying the fibres inserted into the ischial tuberosity, the sciatic nerve is only secondary to the obturator innervation. The obturator nerve is the nerve supply to all the adductor group of muscles including gracilis.

61. The patella

   A   is a sesamoid bone formed from elastic tissue
   B   has articular surfaces divided into a broad medial and narrow lateral areas
   C   receives a tendon from the vastus medialis
   D   begins to ossify soon after puberty
   E   is rarely dislocated medially

62. The popliteal fossa

   A   is a diamond-shaped region behind the knee
   B   has a roof formed by the fascia lata
   C   is limited laterally by the semimembranosus and semitendinosus tendons
   D   has the popliteal artery placed superficially
   E   contains lymph nodes draining the skin of the dorsum of the foot

NEUROLOGY

63. The pons

   A   has the trigeminal nuclei in its middle part
   B   has a posterior surface which contributes to the roof of the fourth ventricle
   C   has a tegmental part which contains the nuclei of the trigeminal, abducent and facial nerves
   D   contains the trapezoid body, and medial longitudinal bundle near the midline
   E   contains the dorsal vagal nucleus and the olivary nucleus

64. Sympathetic nerve fibres

   A   are carried by all spinal nerves
   B   are vasodilators
   C   innervate arrectores pilorum
   D   are from a cranio-sacral outflow
   E   arise from the lateral horns of most cervical segments

Answers overleaf

61. E

The patella, the largest sesamoid bone, is formed from hyaline cartilage and usually begins to ossify at about 3-4 years old. The quadriceps femoris muscles insert into the quadriceps tendon which then inserts into the superior patellar border. The vastus medialis muscle, however, has a muscular insertion with horizontal fibres to resist the natural tendency of the patella to dislocate laterally. The shape of the articular surface is also designed to resist this dislocation, a vertical ridge dividing the articular surface into a narrow medial and broad lateral area.

62. A B

The popliteal fossa is limited above and medially by the semimembranosus and semitendinosus and laterally by the biceps tendon. In the fossa the nerves lie the most superficially, then the popliteal vein and most deeply placed lies the popliteal artery. This explains the difficulty in finding the popliteal pulse even in the normal healthy person. The lymphatics of the skin on the dorsum of the foot drain along a similar course to that of the long saphenous vein towards the superficial inguinal lymph nodes. The lymph nodes in the fossa are draining the heel and the foot and a small area along the calf, i.e. the approximate drainage area of the short saphenous vein.

63. A C D

The posterior pontine surface contributes to the floor, not the roof of the fourth ventricle. As well as the nuclei of the Vth, VIth and VIIth nerves, the vestibulocochlear (VIIIth) nerve nuclei are also contained in the tegmental part of the pons. The trapezoid body is the crossed axons of the cochlear nuclei whilst the medial longitudinal bundle connects head, eye and neck movements to sounds. Both the dorsal vagal nucleus and the olivary nucleus are found at the level of the open medulla, caudal to the pons.

64. A C

The sympathetics are derived from the lateral horns of the T1-L2 spinal cord segments. There is no cervical nor sacral sympathetic outlfow. Cranio-sacral autonomic outflow is from the parasympathetics. The sympathetics are vasoconstrictors.

65. The middle cerebral artery

A lies within the insula
B supplies all the motor and sensory cerebral areas for the opposite half of the body
C supplies the speech area of Broca
D reaches the lateral surface of the hemisphere via the lateral fissure
E supplies the superior frontal gyrus

66. Transection of the cervical sympathetic chain produces

A dilatation of the pupil
B ptosis
C exophthalmos
D ipsilateral facial sweating
E ipsilateral flushing of the face

67. Thrombosis of the posterior inferior cerebellar artery causes

A speech impairment (dysphonia)
B loss of pain and temperature sensation on the same side of the face
C loss of pain and temperature sensation on the opposite side of the body
D palatal palsy
E double vision (diplopia)

68. The spinal cord

A possesses two symmetrical enlargements which correspond to the limb plexuses
B extends lower in the adult than in the fetus
C is supplied mainly by the anterior and posterior spinal arteries
D has a central mass of white matter enclosed in a cylinder of grey matter
E supplies the thyrohyoid and geniohyoid muscles from the 1st cervical nerve

Answers overleaf

65. A C D

The middle cerebral artery passes into the lateral sulcus and crosses the temporal lobe and insula, eventually reaching the lateral surface of the hemisphere. It supplies the motor and sensory cerebral areas for the opposite half of the body excluding the leg, perineum and auditory centre. The superior frontal gyrus is supplied by the anterior cerebral artery.

66. B E

Cervical chain transection causes a loss of control of the dilator pupillae and so the pupil constricts. Exophthalmos is an outward bulging of the eyeball, whereas, if anything, enophthalmos is said to occur in sympathetic chain lesions. Due to the lack of sudomotor control there is little or no sweating on the ipsilateral side, and loss of blood vessel control causes increased vascularisation and flushing.

67. A B C D

A posterior inferior cerebellar artery (P.I.C.A.) thrombosis causes infarction of the nucleus ambiguus and so paralysis of the semi-abducted vocal cord making normal speech difficult. Damage to the uncrossed spinal tract of V gives same side loss of pain and temperature whereas the loss on the opposite side is due to the crossed spinal lemniscus. A palatal palsy is due to bulbar palsy. Vision is not affected as the visual tracts and nuclei involved in vision are lying cephalad in the midbrain and upper pons.

68. A C E

The cervical and lumbar enlargements correspond to the limb plexi. In the fetus, the spinal cord often extends to L3, whereas the adult cord usually ends at the L1 or occasionally L2 level. This difference is due to the increased rate of growth of the bony vertebral column during development. The cord has a central mass of grey matter enclosed in white matter (mainly myelinated tracts). Although it looks as if the hypoglossal nerve supplies these muscles, it is just acting as a carrier for C1 nerve fibres in the ansa hypoglossi.

Anatomy

69. Posterior primary rami supply

   A   all trunk muscles
   B   splenius capitis
   C   skin over the calf muscles
   D   upper limb extensor muscles
   E   vertebral column extensors and overlying skin

70. The vagus (X) nerve

   A   has the most extensive distribution of all the cranial nerves
   B   is the main motor and secretor motor nerve to the gut and its glands
   C   supplies the tympanic membrane
   D   is sensory to the thoracic viscera
   E   is motor to the sigmoid colon

HISTOLOGY

71. Smooth muscle fibres

   A   have a single nucleus located centrally
   B   contain just a few striated bands
   C   do not contain thick myosin filaments
   D   possess A and I bands
   E   contain A.T.P. and creatine phosphate in lower concentrations than found in skeletal muscle fibres

72. Cells of the APUD system

   A   can take up amine precursors
   B   contain an amino acid decarboxylase
   C   may secrete gastrin, somatostatin or substance P
   D   have high levels of rough endoplasmic reticulum
   E   include the thyroid C cells

Answers overleaf

69. **B E**

Some of the trunk-musculature posteriorly such as the erector spinae group are supplied by the posterior rami, but trunk muscles such as the abdominals are anterior rami innervated. The muscles and skin of both upper and lower limbs are supplied by the anterior primary rami even on the posterior or extensor surfaces. Posterior primary rami do not supply limbs.

70. **A B C D**

The vagus has a very wide distribution including parasympathetic, special visceral motor, general and special visceral sensory and somatic sensory fibres. The parasympathetic fibres supply the heart, lungs and the gut as far as the splenic flexure. The somatic sensory fibres go to the external acoustic meatus posteriorly, and the tympanic membrane. The sigmoid colon is supplied by parasympathetics from the sacral region.

71. **A E**

In smooth muscle, there is an absence of striated banding patterns in the cytoplasm (hence its name). These bands arise from the arrangement of the myosin thick filaments and the actin thin filaments as seen in striated muscle. In smooth muscle, however, these filaments are distributed throughout the cytoplasm, orientated parallel to the fibre but not organised into regular units of filaments. At high magnification, the thick filaments can be seen to possess cross bridges, just as in skeletal muscle.

72. **A B C E**

APUD stands for (A) contains a fluorogenic amine or at least can secondarily take it up. (PU) can take up amine precursors, e.g. DOPA, i.e. Precursor Uptake. (D) contains an amino acid Decarboxylase. The cells of the APUD cell system have low levels of rough endoplasmic reticulum. This is not truly specific to the APUD system cells, but seen in most protein-secreting cells. Many of the APUD peptides such as gastrin, somatostatin VIP etc. have been isolated not only in the gut, but have also now been isolated from the brain.

73. **A stained preparation has a true ciliated border and smooth muscle fibres. This section could have been taken from the**

    A   vas deferens
    B   fimbriae of the oviduct
    C   epiglottis
    D   small respiratory bronchioles
    E   upper lobe bronchus

74. **Cartilage**

    A   contains a matrix which consists of ground substance and connective tissue fibres
    B   is always surrounded by perichondrium even at the articular surfaces
    C   contains chondrocytes which lie within small smooth-walled lacunae
    D   matrix has a low content of chondroitin sulphate
    E   rarely contains elastic fibres

75. **In the digestive system, the**

    A   serous glands (Von Ebner) of the tongue are located in the region of the vallate papilae
    B   chief and parietal cells are found mainly near the cardia and pylorus
    C   Brunner's glands are found in the jejunum
    D   appendix does not contain any crypts of Lieberkuhn
    E   parotid gland is purely serous

EMBRYOLOGY

76. **The structures derived from the first pharyngeal arch are the**

    A   stapes footplate
    B   malleus
    C   stylohoid ligament
    D   incus
    E   greater horn of the hyoid bone

Answers overleaf

73. B E

Normal respiratory epithelium such as seen in the bronchus and bronchioles is ciliated pseudostratified columnar epithelium. In the smaller respiratory bronchioles however, the cells are low columnar or cuboidal and the cilia have disappeared. The vas and epididymis have pseudostratified columnar cells with a border of stereocilia which under E.M. are shown to lack the true structural characteristics of cilia. They are, in fact, very long microvilli. The epiglottis is, of course, a classical site of elastic cartilage and does not contain a ciliated border.

74. A C

Perichondrium is a layer of irregular fibrous connective tissue which always invests hyaline cartilage except at the free surfaces of articular cartilage. The matrix, in hyaline cartilage, is composed of ground substance (protein polysaccharide) and connective tissue fibres and has a very high chondroitin sulphate content often seen as metachromasia when stained with toluidine blue. Cartilage does not only refer to the ubiquitous hyaline cartilage, but there is, of course, elastic cartilage with abundant elastic fibres such as seen in the epiglottis.

75. A E

The gastric mucosa, containing the chief cells, which secrete pepsinogen and mucoproteins, and the parietal cells secreting HCl, is found throughout most of the stomach except for the cardiac and pyloric regions. Brunner's glands (first described by Wepfer, Brunner's father-in-law) are diagnostic of the duodenum. They are compound tubular and are composed of low columnar cells which secrete mucus. The histology of the appendix resembles that of the colon and therefore as well as the crypts contains numerous lymph nodules and has a submucosa rich in fat cells.

76. B D

The structures derived from the first pharyngeal arch are the malleus, incus, the sphenomandibular ligament and Meckel's cartilage. The stapes, styloid and stylohyoid ligament as far as the lesser cornu (horn) are all derived from the second arch and the greater horn of the hyoid bone is derived from the third arch cartilage.

77. In the normal development of the female genital tract, the

A lower part of the vagina is formed from the sinovaginal bulbs

B upper vagina is formed from the fused mesonephric ducts

C round ligament of the uterus is formed from the paramesonephric duct

D greater vestibular glands (Bartholin) are outgrowths from the urogenital sinus

E vaginal lumen is separated from the urogenital sinus by the pectinate line

78. In the fetal circulation, the

A septum secundum contains no foramen

B obliterated part of the umbilical arteries become the ligamentum teres of the adult

C umbilical vein drains into the ductus venosus

D pressure in the right atrium is slightly higher than that of the left atrium

E ductus venosus connects the right umbilical vein with the right hepatocardiac vein

79. In the developing digestive system, the

A biliary apparatus is a midgut derivative

B Kupffer cells are derived from the splanchnic mesenchyme of the septum transversum

C liver is a major site of haemopoiesis during the second month

D bulk of the pancreas is derived from the ventral bud

E area of fusion of the urorectal septum with the cloacal membrane becomes the trigone of the bladder

80. In the normal five week embryo, disease processes are likely to affect normal development of the

A heart

B central nervous system

C external genitalia

D teeth

E ear

Answers overleaf

77. A D

The upper vagina is formed by the fused paramesonephric ducts whilst the ovarian ligament and round ligament of the uterus are derived from the gubernaculum ovarii. The proctodeum and cloaca of the rectum are separated by the pectinate line, whereas the vaginal lumen and urogenital sinus are divided by a membrane called the hymen which usually ruptures during the perinatal period.

78. C

The septum secundum of the atria has a foramen so that the septum primum can act as a flap-valve between the atria. The blood from the placenta travels via the left umbilical vein to the ductus venosus which connects with the right hepatocardiac vein and on to the inferior vena cava. The ligamentum venosum of the adult is the obliterated ductus venosus and the left umbilical vein becomes the ligamentum teres of the adult. In the fetus, the right and left atrial pressures are equal.

79. B C

The biliary apparatus and liver are foregut derivatives and although the pancreas does develop from both ventral and dorsal mesentry, it is the dorsal bud which forms the bulk of the adult organ. The ventral bud forms part of the head and uncinate process of the pancreas. The region of fusion between urorectal septum and the cloacal membrane gives rise to the perineal body, the major anchor-point of the perineal musculature of special clinical significance in post-partum women.

80. A B E

Development of the embryo is most easily disturbed during organogenesis particularly from day 13 to day 60. During this time, disease processes or teratogenic agents may be lethal or cause major morphological abnormalities. Each organ has a critical period during which its development may be deranged. The central nervous system is vulnerable from 2 weeks onwards, particularly until 6 weeks, the heart from 3-6 weeks and the ear from 4-10 weeks. These three organs are therefore particularly sensitive at 5 weeks. The teeth, however, are later in development from 6-10 weeks as are the external genitalia from 7 weeks onwards. These would therefore be spared should a problem arise in a five week old embryo.

PHYSIOLOGY

CARDIOVASCULAR AND BLOOD

81. Plasma proteins

    A on electrophoresis migrate at different rates to the anode and cathode

    B contribute largely to the osmotic pressure of plasma

    C concentration falls early in starvation

    D are involved in the transport of thyroid, adrenocortical and gonadal hormones

    E are responsible for 15% of the buffering capacity of the blood

82. Loss of fluid from the capillaries is

    A decreased by arteriolar constriction

    B decreased by venoconstriction

    C increased by accumulation of osmotically active substances in the interstitial space

    D increased in heart failure

    E decreased when the plasma protein concentration is reduced

83. Lymph

    A clots on standing

    B usually contains more protein than plasma

    C does not contain cells

    D conveys certain enzymes into the circulation

    E daily flow is about 1 litre

84. Platelets

    A are cell fragments in blood

    B help overcome infection

    C are present in numbers of 7×10^9 cells/litre blood

    D are important in blood clotting

    E are usually produced in the spleen

Answers overleaf

81. A D E

Plasma protein concentration is maintained in starvation. The osmotic pressure of plasma proteins plays an important role in the exchange of fluid across the capillaries, but is only 25mm/Hg which represents a small proportion of the total osmotic pressure of plasma. Electophoretic mobility is the basis of separation of plasma proteins. In addition to serving as binding proteins for certain hormones, they contribute to the buffering capacity of blood.

82. A C

Arteriolar constriction produces reduced capillary pressure and net movement of fluid into the vascular compartment. Venoconstriction in contrast, causes increased capillary fluid loss as does an increase in venous pressure occurring in heart failure. The osmotic gradient is also important in the formation of tissue fluid; increases in the osmotic pressure of the interstitial tissue and reduced plasma protein both lead to increased loss of capillary fluid.

83. A D

The protein content of the lymph varies with the organ from which the lymph drains, but, in general, is lower than that of the plasma. The proteins do, however, include clotting factors, and certain enzymes such as lipase and histaminase, which enter the circulation via the lymphatics. Lymphocytes reach the circulation through the lymphatics and relatively large numbers are present in the thoracic duct. The normal lymph flow over 24 hours is about 2-4 litres.

84. A D

Platelets are cell fragments in the blood, lacking nuclei, and are derived from megakaryocytes in the bone marrow. They are destroyed in the spleen. They are important in blood clotting, but have no role in overcoming infection, which is a function of the leucocytes. A count of 7×10^9 cells/litre blood is also characteristic of leucocytes. Platelets are present in numbers of 250×10^{12}/litre blood.

85. In transfusing blood

A heparin is used as the anticoagulant
B it should be stored at 0° c
C a person over 15 years may be a habitual donor
D group 0 subjects are universal donors
E group AB subjects are universal donors

86. An increased prothrombin time (PT)

A can be restored to normal by the administration of
 protamine
B occurs occasionally in jaundice
C is seen in patients taking the anticoagulant coumarin
D may be seen after a blood transfusion
E is seen in patients given heparin

87. The haemoglobin-oxygen dissociation curve is shifted to the left by

A fever
B metabolic acidosis
C erythropoietin
D anaemia
E chronic hypoxia

88. The effects of whole blood loss are

A an immediate reduction in the haematocrit
B widespread venoconstriction
C contraction of the spleen
D constriction of efferent and afferent arterioles
E an increase in aldosterone secretion

Answers overleaf

Physiology

85. D

In obtaining blood for transfusion it should be stored at 4° c, citrate being used as the anticoagulant. It would be inadvisable to accept as a habitual donor someone still growing. Group 0 subjects are universal donors and group AB subjects universal recipients.

86. B C

The prothrombin test gives an estimate of the extrinsic system, whereas heparin inhibits the action of thrombin. Protamine only neutralizes heparin. Many clotting factors may be abnormal in liver disease or obstructive jaundice. Oral anticoagulants such as dicoumarin competitively inhibit vitamin K. Citrate which is used in stored blood bonds calcium, so, with a large transfusion, there may be a Ca^{++} deficiency. However, Ca^{++} is part of the intrinsic pathway, and so this does not affect the prothrombin time.

87. All false

A shift of the haemoglobin dissociation curve to the left means that for any given pO_2 the haemoglobin has a greater affinity for oxygen. Increased temperature and increased arterial acidity shift the haemoglobin curve to the right. Erythropoietin stimulates red cell production, but does not affect their capacity to carry oxygen.

88. B D E

A wide variety of compensatory mechanisms are brought into play in haemorrhage. There is a reduced renal plasma flow with decreased GFR and urine flow. There is increased sodium absorption under the influence of aldosterone. There is widespread venoconstriction which serves to increase venous return. The haematocrit is maintained for a number of hours after the start of bleeding, but this is not a result of contraction of the spleen which does not occur in man.

89. Heart rate is increased by

A   increased intracranial pressure
B   inspiration
C   assumption of the upright from the lying posture
D   adrenaline
E   stimulation of pain fibres in the trigeminal nerve

90. During the cardiac cycle

A   diastole always lasts longer than systole
B   the right and left ventricles contract at the same time
C   the onset of ventricular contraction is synchronous with the P wave of the ECG
D   atrial pressure rises during isovolumetric relaxation
E   atrial contraction accounts for 50% of ventricular filling

91. The sinu-atrial node

A   is situated at the right atrium close to the coronary sinus
B   has a conduction rate equal to that of the AV node
C   is depressed by digitalis
D   is innervated chiefly by the left vagus
E   contains rhythmically discharging cells which have a variable rate of discharge

92. Cardiac output

A   can be measured by the direct Fick method
B   at rest is approximately 5 l/min
C   can only be altered by changes in heart rate
D   is related to venous return
E   at rest is ¼ of maximum

Answers overleaf

89. B C D

Increased intracranial pressure and stimulation of pain fibres in the trigeminal nerve both depress the heart rate. In children and young adults, heart rate speeds on inspiration, a process called sinus arrhythmia. On assumption of the upright posture, there is a redistribution of blood with some venous pooling and a reflex increase in heart rate which helps maintain blood pressure. Catecholamines have a direct chronotropic effect on the heart, but the accompanying pressor response of noradrenaline produces a reflex bradycardia.

90. D

When the heart rate is increased, as in exercise, systole may be longer than diastole. Atrial contraction accounts for no more than 30% of ventricular filling. The left ventricle contracts first, the onset of contraction being mirrored in the QRS complex, the P wave corresponding to atrial contraction. During the isovolumetric relaxation phase of contraction, atrial pressure rises.

91. C E

The sinu-atrial (SA) node is situated near the right auricular appendage, and is innervated by the right vagus. An effect similar to that of vagal stimulation is produced by digitalis. Like other parts of the conduction system, the cells discharge spontaneously, but the SA node discharges most rapidly. It also has the fastest rate of conduction.

92. A B D

The Fick principle, when applied to determination of cardiac output by a consideration of oxygen becomes

$$CO = \frac{O_2 \text{ uptake in ml/min}}{A\text{-}V \ O_2 \text{ difference}} \times 100 \text{ mg}$$

The value at rest is 5l/min, and can increase up to 40l/min in exercise. The value is related to venous return and can be increased by increases in heart rate and stroke volume.

93. Circulation of blood through the brain

A   is uniform throughout the tissue
B   is independent of intracranial pressure
C   is on average 100ml/100g/min in adults
D   is increased by a fall in the pH of extracellular fluid
E   is affected by marked gravitational changes

94. Myocardial contractility is depressed by

A   sympathetic stimulation
B   alkalosis
C   procaineamide
D   digoxin
E   hypercapnia

95. Dilation of the arterioles can be induced by

A   a fall in local temperature
B   histamine
C   a fall in pCO_2
D   decreased adrenergic discharge
E   increased angiotensin II concentrations

RESPIRATION

96. The affinity of haemoglobin for oxygen is

A   decreased by alkalosis
B   decreased by increasing body temperature
C   increased by increasing concentrations of 2, 3 diphosphoglycerate
D   decreased by serotonin
E   decreased by hypoxia

Answers overleaf

93. D

Blood flow through various brain tissues varies, being relatively high in the cortex. Blood flow distribution also depends on the activity of the individual. Flow decreases with intracranial pressure and there is compensation for changes in arterial pressure at the level of the head, as for example, in situations of altered gravitational field. Vasomoter reflexes play little if any part in regulation of the cerebral circulation. Flow is influenced by brain metabolism so that an increase in hydrogen ion concentration can be accompanied by an increase in blood flow.

94. C E

Myocardial contractility is depressed by a number of factors including hypercapnia, procaineamide and acidosis. It is increased by digoxin and by sympathetic stimulation which induces an increased movement of calcium into the cytosol during excitation.

95. B D

Arteriolar constriction results from a fall in local temperature. It is also produced by angiotensin II, which is a very powerful agent giving an increase in blood pressure. Vasodilation is produced by a number of agents including histamine and a rise in pCO_2. Adrenergic discharge keeps the smooth muscle in the arteriolar wall in a state of partial contraction. Decreased adrenergic discharge therefore results in dilation.

96. B

Carriage of oxygen by haemoglobin is influenced by a number of factors. With increasing carbon dioxide tension and hydrogen ion concentration, more oxygen is released into a given tissue, i.e. the affinity is decreased. Increase in temperature has a similar effect, so that in more active tissues. more oxygen is given off. Another important factor influencing the affinity of haemoglobin for oxygen is the concentration of 2, 3 diphosphoglycerate (2, 3 DPG), increasing concentrations leading to a reduced affinity. The percent saturation of haemoglobin is influenced by oxygen tension, but not affinity. Serotonin has no effect.

97. After exercise, the oxygen debt

A may be six times basal oxygen consumption
B in trained athletes is greater than in an untrained person for a given amount of exercise
C is limited by an increase in pH
D is increased because blood cannot be delivered to the muscles at a fast enough rate
E is possible because the muscle is capable of anaerobic metabolism

98. Inhalation of 5% CO_2 at normal atmospheric pressure

A produces bradycardia
B decreases alveolar ventilation
C produces a fall in blood pH
D reduces the partial pressure of oxygen in the lungs
E reduces the pH of the cerebrospinal fluid

99. Carbon dioxide is carried in the circulation

A at a partial pressure of 46 mmHg in venous blood
B at a partial pressure of 100 mmHg
C in association with amino groups
D largely in red blood cells
E largely as carbonic acid

100. Airways resistance is

A inversely proportional to the airways radius
B directly proportional to length
C increased by histamine
D greater in expiration than inspiration
E decreased in response to stimulation of irritant receptors

97. A D E

The oxygen debt can be six times basal oxygen consumption indicating that it allows a greater degree of exertion than would otherwise be possible. Trained athletes produce a smaller oxygen debt for a given amount of exertion, as they are able to increase the oxygen consumption of their muscles to a greater degree. The oxygen debt is possible because of anaerobic metabolism. Lactic acid is formed so that there is a fall in pH which is rate limiting.

98. C E

If the inspired CO_2 is increased, there is an increase in the hydrogen ion concentration in both blood and cerebrospinal fluid (CSF), due to the formation of carbonic acid, which dissociates into hydrogen and bicarbonate ions. The changes in the pH of the CSF result in stimulation of respiration. There is no effect on the partial pressure of oxygen in the lungs.

99. A C E

The partial pressure of CO_2 in venous blood is about 46 mmHg. Some is carried in the red cell and in combination with amino groups of proteins, principally haemoglobin. The largest fraction is carried in solution. However, the actual amount as carbonic acid is relatively small as it ionizes to bicarbonate.

100. B C D E

Airways resistance is directly proportional to the length of the airways and inversely proportional to the fourth power of the airway radius. It is greater in expiration than inspiration, and is affected by a number of chemical agents including histamine, which causes constriction of the airways and thus increases airway resistance. It is decreased also in response to stimulation of irritant receptors.

101. The respiratory centre may be stimulated directly or indirectly by

A the partial pressure of carbon dioxide in blood
B the hydrogen ion concentration in whole blood
C the partial pressure of oxygen
D afferent fibres from proprioceptors
E efferent vagal fibres

102. The functional residual capacity

A is about 1.0 l
B is the volume of gas left in lungs at the resting expiratory level
C is the combined residual volume and inspiratory capacity
D can be determined from analyses of samples of alveolar air
E can be measured with a spirometer

103. Hypoxia

A occurs in anaemic subjects
B may complicate kyphoscoliosis
C is likely to develop with increases in total atmospheric pressure
D affects aortic and carotid baroreceptor cells
E produces polycythaemia

104. Acclimatisation is associated with

A an increase in 2, 3 diphosphoglycerate (2, 3 DPG) in erythrocytes
B an increase in plasma hydrogen ion concentration
C relative anaemia
D increased alveolar PO_2 values
E increase in ventilation

Answers overleaf

101. A B C D

The respiratory centre is stimulated directly by a number of factors including an increase in the carbon dioxide tension and oxygen lack. A fall in PO_2 causes respiratory stimulation via peripheral chemoreceptors, and a rise in PCO_2 stimulates respiration both via peripheral chemoreceptors and centrally via medullary receptors, which respond to H^+ changes in their immediate environment. The main proprioceptor input to the respiratory is from the lungs, but there is also input from the joints and tendons. Afferent, not efferent vagal fibres pass to the centre.

102. B

The functional reserve volume in the healthy adult is about 3.0 l and is a combination of residual volume and expiratory reserve volume, being the volume of air in the lungs at the end of quiet expiration. It cannot be measured using analysis of samples of alveolar air or with a spirometer, but requires dilution of a gas such as nitrogen or helium.

103. A B E

Four types of anoxia are recognised. Anaemic anoxia occurs when there is a reduced amount of haemoglobin for O_2 carriage. Anoxic hypoxia occurs in kyphoscoliosis as deformities of the rib cage reduce ventilation. The other two types are stagnant and histotoxic anaemia. An increase in barometric pressure does not reduce oxygen tensions. Hypoxia results in stimulation of the chemoreceptors, not baroreceptors, but does lead to polycythaemia.

104. A E

Acclimatisation is achieved by a number of compensatory mechanisms including increased alveolar ventilation, with an accompanying fall in plasma hydrogen ion concentrations, an increase in packed cell volume and haemoglobin content, and a shift of the haemoglobin dissociation curve to the right produced by increased 2, 3 DPG production. The concentration of hydrogen ions in the CSF gradually returns to normal. Alveolar PO_2 values are unaltered.

105. **The arterial carbon dioxide tension is determined by**

    A alveolar ventilation
    B carbon dioxide transfer from blood to alveoli
    C ventilation/perfusion ratio
    D the level of 2, 3 diphosphoglycerate
    E lung compliance

106. **Surfactant in the lung**

    A is a phospholipoprotein complex
    B when deficient results in respiratory distress in the
        newborn
    C maturation of synthetic mechanisms is facilitated by
        cortisol
    D reduces surface tension in all the alveoli to the
        same degree
    E prevents small alveoli collapsing into larger

METABOLISM

107. **Iodine is**

    A absorbed as iodide
    B ingested in approximate daily quantities of 500 mg
    C excreted only by the kidneys
    D is actively transported to the choroid plexus
    E is firmly bound to protein in the thyroid

108. **In the course of iron metabolism**

    A 3-6% of dietary iron is normally absorbed
    B most of the iron is absorbed in the stomach
    C iron absorption is inhibited by pancreatic juice
    D on average, men and women lose about 108 μmol iron
        per day
    E 70% of the iron in the body is incorporated into haemoglobin

Answers overleaf

105. A C E

The depth of alveolar ventilation influences carbon dioxide tension, hyperventilation producing a drop in pCO_2. The ventilation perfusion ratio also affects pCO_2 but a reduction in the transfer of CO_2 sufficient to cause CO_2 retention would be incompatible with life. In disease states with decreased compliance chronic elevation of pCO_2 is found concentrations of 2, 3 diphosphoglycerate affect O_2 transport.

106. A B C E

Surfactant is a phospholipoprotein and is believed to be produced by type II alveolar cells. Insufficient surfactant in the newborn results in respiratory distress syndrome. Maturation of the synthetic mechanisms is facilitated by cortisol, administration of which, to pregnant women, combats disease in premature infants. The importance of surfactant is that it prevents smaller alveoli collapsing into larger, an effect not achieved were surface tension altered in all alveoli to the same degree.

107. A D E

About 500 μg iodine are taken in daily. It is converted to iodide in the gastrointestinal tract in which from it is absorbed. It is excreted both by the kidneys and the gastrointestinal tract. Iodine is actively taken up into a number of tissues other than the thyroid gland.

108. A C E

Only 3-6% of dietary iron is absorbed and this occurs in the upper part of the small intestine. The stomach does play a role in the absorption in that gastric secretions dissolve iron, and reduce it to the ferrous form. The greatest part of iron–70%–is in haemoglobin, 3% in myoglobin and the remainder in ferritin. Men lose 108 μmol iron per day, but women lose twice this amount.

109. The serum cholesterol concentration

    A is lowered by clofibrate
    B falls if a low cholesterol diet is taken
    C rises with a diet high in saturated fats
    D rises in mild thyrotoxicosis
    E falls with biliary obstruction

110. Under normal circumstances, phosphate

    A absorption may be prevented by aluminium hydroxide ingestion
    B deficiency may give symptons of muscle weakness
    C concentrations in the plasma are 3.9 mmol/1
    D exists in both the organic and inorganic form in the plasma
    E deficiency is caused by increased renal excretion

111. Hyponatreamia may accompany

    A cancer of the lung
    B renal disease
    C Addison's disease
    D congestive heart failure
    E the use of frusemide (Lasix)

112. Within the body, potassium

    A is mainly in the intracellular compartment
    B concentrations in plasma are a good indicator of total body potassium
    C is not absorbed in the proximal tubule
    D loss in the urine is increased by spironolactone
    E in raised concentrations (hyperkalaemia) causes a tenting of the T wave in the ECG

Answers overleaf

Physiology

109. **A B C**

Clofibrate is used therapeutically to reduce serum cholesterol. The concentrations also fall in mild thyrotoxicosis, and if a low cholestrol diet is taken, even though synthesis does increase to some extent in this instance. Serum cholesterol concentrations rise with a diet high in saturated fats and with biliary obstruction.

110. **A B C D E**

About 1-1.5 g dietary phosphate are required daily. Normally, this requirement is easily met, but, if for example the antacid aluminium hydroxide is taken in excess, the insoluble aluminium phosphate is formed with resultant deficiency symptoms such as muscle weakness. Deficiency may also result from impaired renal reabsorption. The plasma phosphate comprises 2.8 mmol organic phosphate and 1.1 mmol inorganic phosphate.

111. **A C**

Occasionally, a carcinoma of the lung may synthesise hormones including vasopressin (ADH) and this leads to the Schwartz Barrter syndrome, (SIADH) characterised by the production of a relatively concentrated urine in the face of a reduced plasma sodium. Patients with renal disease and congestive heart failure tend to retain sodium. Water retention and sodium loss are also seen in adrenal insufficiency. Potassium is the main ion lost with frusemide administration.

112. **A E**

The sodium and chloride ions in the body are largely confined to the extracellular fluid, the potassium ions to the intracellular compartment, so that the plasma potassium concentration is not a very good indicator of total body potassium. Potassium can be absorbed by the proximal tubule, and can be secreted into the urine in the distal tubule, a process influenced by aldosterone. Spironolactone is an antagonist of the action of aldosterone and so produces a loss of sodium in the urine. In the presence of elevated potassium concentrations, the T waves become tall and peaked as a result of altered repolarisation.

113. **Calcium**

    A   increases the excitability of the neuromuscular junction
    B   increases the contractility of cardiac muscle fibres
    C   is necessary for normal blood clotting
    D   has serum concentrations raised by a thyroid extract
    E   is not bound to protein in the plasma

114. **Vitamin B₁₂**

    A   is a cobalt containing substance
    B   deficiency causes large primitive red cell precursors to
        appear in the peripheral plasma
    C   is mainly absorbed in the stomach
    D   is bound firmly to intrinsic factor prior to absorption
    E   deficiency is usually due to inadequate dietary intake

115. **The pH of arterial blood is decreased by**

    A   hyperventilation
    B   a right to left shunt
    C   a uretero-colic anastomosis
    D   diabetic ketosis
    E   ammonium chloride ingestion

116. **Magnesium deficiency**

    A   may accompany convulsions especially in babies
    B   may occur during intravenous feeding
    C   is necessary for the breakdown of ATP
    D   is indicated by a serum magnesium of 1 mmol/1
    E   gives rise to peripheral vasodilatation

Answers overleaf

113. A B C

Calcium ions have a marked influence on excitable tissue, adequate concentrations also being required for the release of acetyl choline at the muscle end-plate. Calcium is important in blood clotting, acting at several stages in the cascade process. An extract of thyroid gland would contain calcitonin, which acts to lower serum calcium concentrations. Not all blood calcium exists in the free form; nearly half is protein bound.

114. A B D

The term vitamin B_{12} describes a number of cobalamine compounds, a deficiency of which causes megaloblastic anaemia. Vitamin B_{12} is largely absorbed in the terminal ileum, a process requiring intrinsic factor. Deficiency usually results from defective absorption, although dietary deficiency is not uncommon in strict vegetarians.

115. C D E

Unless there is some other respiratory or metabolic disturbance, there should be no alteration in acid-base status in patients with a left to right shunt. Hyperventilation reduces pCO_2 and hence increases pH. With uretero-colic anastomoses, there is hydrogen ion absorption from the colon. Both ketones and ammonium chloride yield hydrogen ions.

116. A B C

Magnesium deficiency is frequently accompanied by changes in serum calcium and hence convulsions. Deficiency could occur during prolonged intravenous feeding in which case the addition of trace elements would be required. A value of 1 mmol for the serum concentration is in the normal range. Peripheral vasodilatation is a sign of magnesium excess, not deficiency.

Physiology

GASTROENTEROLOGY

117. The malabsorption syndrome

A does not usually occur after removal of a short segment of
jejunum or ileum
B may result in bleeding tendencies
C may reduce the quantity of fat in the faeces
D may present with oedema
E does not occur in tropical sprue and coeliac disease

118. The secretion of saliva

A is hormonally controlled
B results mainly from conditioned reflexes
C follows stimulation of the chorda tympani
D is necessary for complete digestion of starch
E provides antiseptic protection of the mouth

119. In the course of carbohydrate digestion and absoprtion

A carbohydrates are initially attacked by salivary amylase
B sucrose is split to form glucose and galactose
C glucose enters the portal circulation by passive transport
D trypsin hydrolyses the 1-4-α linkages of the carbohydrates
E absorption of sugars is influenced by Na^+

120. The hormone gastrin

A is produced in cells that appear to be of neural crest origin
B is not secreted in significant amounts in the duodenum
C may exist in more than one molecular form
D stimulates insulin and glucagon secretion
E has its secretion reduced by atropine

Answers overleaf

59

Physiology

117. A B D

In the malabsorption syndrome, there is reduced fat absorption so that a greater quantity appears in the faeces. There is also a failure to reabsorb vitamin K and therefore a reduction in prothrombin production. The failure to absorb amino acids leads to hypoproteinaemia and oedema. The syndrome does occur in tropical sprue and coeliac disease, but not after removal of short segments of the intestine.

118. C E

Salivary secretion is not under hormonal control but the gland receives both sympathetic and parasympathetic nerve supplies. Important stimuli for salivary secretion are taste and mastication. Although it contains the enzyme amylase it contributes little to digestion. Amongst the several functions it provides is antiseptic protection of the mouth.

119. A E

Amylase acts on starch to form disaccharides and trisaccharides. Sucrose is broken down to fructose and glucose which enters the portal circulation by active transport, a process influenced by Na^+. Trypsin is involved in the digestion of proteins.

120. A C D

In common with other hormones of the gastrointestinal tract, gastrin is secreted by cells of neural origin. It is produced by cells of the gastric antrum, and also by the duodenum. It occurs in several molecular forms. In addition to stimulating gastric secretion, it stimulates insulin and glucagon after a protein meal. Atropine, even though it is a cholinergic antagonist, increases gastric secretion.

121. Primary megacolon

   A is due to the absence of myenteric ganglion cells
   B mainly affects adults
   C may be treated surgically
   D may be associated with urinary tract anomalies
   E mainly affects the distal colon

122. The gastro-intestinal tract hormone cholecystokinin-pancreozymin

   A stimulates gastric emptying
   B causes contraction of the gall bladder
   C stimulates glucagon secretion
   D is secreted in response to fatty acids in the duodenum
   E possesses five terminal amino acids identical to gastrin

123. Following total gastrectomy

   A vitamin B_{12} should be administered parenterally
   B lack of pepsin results in abnormal protein digestion
   C iron deficiency may occur
   D hypoglycaemia symptoms may occur about 2 hours after a meal
   E there is a fall in plasma volume after a meal contributing to the dumping syndrome

124. In Europeans, gallstones

   A consist mainly of calcium bilirubinate
   B made of cholesterol may be dissolved by chenodeoxycholic acid
   C when caught in the cystic duct will cause profound obstructive jaundice
   D when blocking the common bile duct will give rise to bilirubin in the urine
   E are associated with reduced alkaline-phosphatase

Answers overleaf

Physiology

121. A C D E

Very infrequent bowel movements associated with few symptoms is seen in children with aganglionic megacolon. The condition may be treated by resection of the aganglionic region. Nearly half the patients with this condition have dilated bladders and 4% have dilated ureters, so that there may be some impairment of nervous control of the urinary tract.

122. B C D E

Cholecystokinin-pancreozymin was originally thought to be two separate hormones, one producing contraction of the gall bladder, and the other stimulating pancreatic secretion. It possesses five terminal amino acids identical to gastrin and is secreted in response to a number of factors including the presence of fatty acids in the duodenum. Other actions are to inhibit gastric emptying and to stimulate glucagon secretion.

123. A C D E

After total gastrectomy, the source of intrinsic factor necessary for vitamin B_{12} absorption is lost, so that B_{12} must be administered. Iron deficiency may also occur. Ingesting a meal may be associated with the dumping syndrome. Glucose rapidly enters the intestine causing initially hyperglycaemia and then hypoglycaemia, as a result of stimulating insulin release, and there is rapid entry of a hypertonic solution into the intestine, so water moves into the gut causing a fall in plasma volume. Protein digestion is normal.

124. B C D

In Europeans, gallstones are generally made of cholesterol. The bile duct or hepatic duct must be blocked to produce a definite obstructive jaundice. Patients with obstructive jaundice have bilirubin in the urine and a raised serum alkaline phosphatase is found.

125. Secretion of gastric acid is

    A increased by acidification of the duodenum
    B reduced by cholecystokinin
    C reduced by H₂ blocking drugs
    D increased by histamine
    E reduced by pentagastrin

126. In the digestion and absorption of fat

    A 50% of the triglycerides of the diet are absorbed as monoglycerides
    B the fate of fatty acids does not depend on their size
    C absorption is greatest in the lower parts of the intestine
    D digestion starts in the stomach
    E 5% of the dietary fat is found in the stools.

ENDOCRINOLOGY AND REPRODUCTION

127. Insulin

    A increases uptake of glucose into skeletal muscles
    B decreases glycogen synthesis
    C lowers intracellular potassium concentrations
    D increases fatty acid synthesis in adipose tissue
    E stimulates gastric acid secretion

128. Goitre

    A can develop with iodine deficiency
    B can develop with iodine excess
    C can occur in vegetarians
    D never occurs in Hashimoto's disease
    E occasionally extends behind the sternum into the anterior mediastinum

Answers overleaf

Physiology

125. B C

The passage of acid into the duodenum decreases gastric acid secretion. Cholecystokinin-pancreozymin inhibits gastric acid as does cimetidine (H_2 receptor blocking drug). Stimulation of acid secretion by histamine is the basis of the augmented histamine test. Pentagastrin, an analogue of gastrin, stimulates gastric acid.

126. A E

Fat digestion starts in the duodenum under the influence of pancreatic lipase, fat absorption being greatest in the upper parts of the small intestine. About 50% of the triglycerides are absorbed as monoglycerides. Fatty acids with less than 10-12 carbon atoms pass directly from the mucosal cells to the portal blood. Acids with longer chains are re-esterified to triglycerides. If the diet contains an average amount of fat, 95% will be absorbed.

127. A D E

Insulin acts to lower blood glucose, stimulating uptake of glucose into cells, particularly muscle and adipose tissue and stimulating glycogen synthesis in the liver. It also affects lipid metabolism, amongst other things increasing fatty acid synthesis in adipose tissue. The gastric acid response to insulin may be used as a test of vagotomy.

128. A B C E

Low iodine concentrations in the diet result in endemic goitre, while high iodine concentrations can depress thyroid function for a while. In addition, Hashimoto's disease causes a form of goitre. Goitrogens can be ingested with vegetables such as cabbage, turnips, etc. Goitre may become retrosternal, but always into the superior anterior mediastinum.

129. Cyclic AMP (adenosine-3, 5-monophosphate)

A is formed from ATP (adenosine-triphosphate)
B mediates the effects of many peptide hormones
C mediates the effects of many steroid hormones
D acts via activation of plasma kinase
E is inhibited by caffeine and theophylline

130. Features of Cushing's syndrome are

A hypotension
B loss of sodium
C wasting and weakness of skeletal muscles
D thin skin with pruple striae
E hirsutism

131. Blood glucose is increased by

A adrenaline
B glucagon
C growth hormone
D aldosterone
E sulphonyl urea derivatives

132. Growth hormone

A has the same structure in all mammalian species
B directly controls the incorporation of sulphate into
     cartilage tissue
C is lactogenic in the human
D is diabetogenic
E increases the size of viscera

Answers overleaf

129. A B D

Cyclic AMP is formed from ATP through the action of the enzyme adenylate cyclase. It mediates the action of most peptide hormones activating plasma kinases. The action is limited by phosphodiesterase which breaks down the cyclic AMP. This enzyme is inhibited by the methylxanthine caffeine and theophylline, so they augment the action of cyclic AMP.

130. C D E

The high circulating concentrations of cortisol which possess mineralocorticoid as well as glucocorticoid activity result in sodium retention which in turn leads to high blood pressure. There is generalised breakdown of protein with wasting of skeletal muscle and thinning of the skin. There are many other changes including hirsutism.

131. A B C

Adrenaline, glucagon and growth hormone all increase blood glucose; adrenaline acts to increase hepatic glucose output, and glucagon also increases hepatic glycogenolysis.
Aldosterone has principally mineralocorticoid activity.
Sulphonyl derivatives stimulate secretion of insulin and hence produce a fall in blood glucose.

132. C D E

The amino acid composition of growth hormone varies with mammalian species. The hormone produces an increase in bone length and the size of soft tissues and viscera. Growth hormone does not produce its effect directly on cartilage but via somatomedin. Growth hormone has an anti-insulin action and hence can be diabetogenic

133. Parathyroid hormone (PTH)

A is a polypeptide
B decreases phosphate excretion in the urine
C acts through stimulation of adenylate cyclase
D is excreted in the urine
E mobilizes Ca++ from bone

134. Arginine vasopressin, the antidiuretic hormone is man

A is produced in the posterior lobe of the pituitary gland
B has its secretion reduced by low plasma osmolality
C may circulate in high concentrations in patients with a low
    plasma osmolality
D has its secretion increased in the post-operative period
E acts by increasing the permeability of the loop of Henle
    to water

135. Oestrogens act to

A increase FSH secretion
B produce growth of axillary and pubic hair in the female
C make the sebaceous glands secrete less fluid
D prime the uterus to oxytocin
E decrease the motility of the Fallopian tube

136. Testosterone

A is secreted by the germinal epithelium of the testes
B is secreted by the Leydig cells
C production is stimulated by prolactin
D stimulates the production of spermatozoa in conjunction
    with other hormones
E decreases LH secretion

Answers overleaf

133. A C D E

PTH is a polypeptide hormone comprising some 84 amino acids. It produces increased plasma calcium concentrations via a number of mechanisms including mobilazation of Ca^{++} from bone. It also has a phosphaturic action due to a decrease in the absorption of phosphate.

134. B C D

Vasopressin is synthesised in cell bodies in the supraoptic and paraventricular nuclei and only released from the posterior pituitary. Secretion is reduced in response to a reduced plasma osmolality but in the Schwartz-Barrter syndrome, vasopressin secretion occurs which is inappropriate for plasma osmolality. Secretion is also enhanced in the post-operative period. The hormone acts to increase the permeability of the collecting duct, not of the loop of Henle.

135. D

Oestrogens exert negative feedback on the anterior pituitary to inhibit FSH release. They prime the uterus to oxytocin, and increase the motility of the Fallopian tubes. Oestrogens act on the sebaceous glands to make the secretions more fluid—hence preventing acne. Growth of axillary and pubic hair in the female is largely due to androgens.

136. B D E

Tertosterone is synthesised in the Leydig cells from cholesterol. The pituitary hormone LH stimulates production of testosterone which in turn inhibits LH secretion. FSH together with androgens maintain spermatogenesis in the testes.

137. The peptide hormone glucagon

A is secreted only by the pancreas
B has lipolytic activity
C stimulates gluconeogenesis
D is glycogenolytic in the muscle
E increases myocardial excitability

UROLOGY

138. In order to be used for determination of renal plasma flow, a substance must

A have a molecular weight greater than 70,000
B be bound to plasma proteins
C be entirely removed from the glomerular filtrate
D be excreted by the renal tubule
E be neither excreted nor reabsorbed by renal tubule cells

139. In the proximal convoluted tubule

A sodium is actively reabsorbed
B potassium ions are secreted
C obligatory reabsorption of water occurs
D PAH is actively secreted
E there is partial reabsorption of glucose

140. The counter current system in the kidney

A produces a high concentration of sodium outside the renal tubule
B requires active transport from the efferent arteriole
C requires active transport of sodium in the descending loop of Henle
D entails the thick ascending portion of the loop of Henle being impermeable to water
E can be inhibited by frusemide

Answers overleaf

137. B C

Glucagon is also produced by cells in the duodenum and stomach. It has a lypolytic action and increases gluconeogenesis from amino acids in the liver. Glucagon is not glycogenolytic in muscle, even though it has such an effect in the liver. Glucagon does not affect myocardial activity, although in large doses it exerts positive inotropic effects.

138. D

To be used in the determination of renal plasma flow, a substance is required which is completely removed from the plasma and excreted into the urine during one passage of the blood through the kidney. It needs to be filtered and so should have a molecular weight of less than 70,000 and should not be bound to plasma proteins. It should also be actively excreted. Such a substance is p-aminohippuric acid (PAH).

139. A C D

Sodium and potassium are actively transported from the glomerular filtrate as it passes down the proximal tubule. The resultant increase in osmolality outside the tubule results in passive movement of water. Sugars and amino acids are completely reabsorbed in the tubule. PAH is excreted by the tubule.

140. A D E

The counter current multiplier system in the kidney produces a high concentration of sodium chloride in the renal interstitium. It is thought that the gradient is set up by the long loops of Henle of the juxtamedullary nephrons and collecting ducts with their associated vasa recta acting as a countercurrent system. Development of the gradient depends on the active transport of chloride ions (followed by Na^+) in the thick part of the ascending loop of Henle and the fact that the ascending part is impermeable to water. Frusemide acts to inhibit chloride reabsorption in the medullary thick ascending loop of Henle.

Physiology

141. An osmotic diuresis can be produced by

A mercurial compounds
B mannitol
C infusion of large amounts of urea
D aldosterone
E lack of vasopressin

142. Secretion of acid by the kidney is usually decreased by

A potassium excess
B increased blood cholesterol concentrations
C reduced serum sodium concentrations
D inhibition of carbonic anhydrase
E increased adrenocortical hormone concentration

143. In the urinary bladder

A there is a smooth muscle, the detrusor muscle, lined by a distensible mucous membrane
B intravesical pressure increases linearly with intravesical volume
C the first urge to void is felt at a volume of 500 ml
D the detrusor muscle is supplied by cholinergic nerves which produce contraction
E the perineal muscles and external sphincter can be contracted voluntarily

144. The glomerular filtrate

A is about 100 litres per day in a normal person
B does not contain substances with a molecular weight greater than 60,000 in a healthy person
C may be estimated by measuring inulin clearance
D may be estimated by measuring PAH clearance
E formation involves some active transport mechanism

Answers overleaf

141. **B C**

An osmotic diuresis occurs if the filtered load of a given solute exceeds the capacity of the cells at the site of absorption. Substances such as mannitol, urea and sucrose act as osmotic diuretics. Diuresis may be produced as a result of administration of mercurial compounds or lack of vasopressin or failure to respond to the hormone, but is not an osmotic diuresis.

142. **A D**

Acid excretion is not affected by blood cholesterol or sodium concentrations, but is inhibited by potassium excess and inhibition of carbonic anhydrase. Aldosterone enhances secretion of hydrogen ions.

143. **A D E**

By the law of Laplace, the bladder is able to accommodate more urine with only a small increase in internal bladder pressure as long as the radius continues to increase. The first urge to void is at a volume of 150 ml. The detrusor muscle is supplied by sympathetic and parasympathetic nerves, cholinergic stimulation producing contraction. The exact mechanism of voluntary urination is not clear, but the perineal muscles and external sphincter can be contracted voluntarily.

144. **A C D**

Even though only about 1500 ml urine are excreted per day, the amount filtered daily is about 180 litres. To be filtered in appreciable quantities, a substance should have a molecular weight below approximately 60,000. However, substances with a higher molecular weight such as albumin are found in small quantities in the urine of healthy subjects. Inulin may be used as a measure of glomerular filtration rate, and PAH of renal plasma flow. The glomerular filtrate is formed by a process of filtration only.

145. Creatinuria occurs in

A children
B pregnancy
C obesity
D thyrotoxicosis
E myopathy

146. In the process of micturition

A when the bladder is empty, the female urethra empties by
   contraction of the bulbocavernosus muscle
B the bladder contributes no inherent contractile activity
C in paraplegics voiding can be initiated by provoking
   a mass reflex
D important control is exerted by the internal sphincter
E sympathetic nerves play an important role

147. Renal blood flow

A may be estimated from inulin clearance
B is about 10-20% of cardiac output
C is reduced in exercise
D is decreased by increased activity in the renal
   sympathetic nerves
E is relatively constant over a wide range of blood pressures

NEUROLOGY

148. The sympathetic nervous system

A contracts the ciliary muscles of the eye
B increases gastrointestinal motility
C constricts bronchiole muscles
D causes constriction of the blood vessels of skin and mucosa
E contracts the bladder detrusor muscle

Answers overleaf

145. A B D E

Creatinuria is observed normally in women during and after pregnancy and childbirth. It is not seen in obesity, but rather in starvation or any condition in which there is extensive muscle breakdown such as thyrotoxicosis and secondary diseases of muscle.

146. C

Only in the male is the urethra emptied by contraction of the bulbocavernosus muscle. The female urethra empties by gravity. The bladder does possess some contractile activity. It has been suggested that the main function of the internal sphincter is to prevent reflux of semen into the bladder. The sympathetic nerves play no role in the process of micturition.

147. C D E

Renal blood flow may be determined from PAH clearance and the haematocrit. It is normally 20-25% of the cardiac output, but may be decreased by exercise when a relatively large proportion passes to the muscles. It is decreased by increased activity in the renal sympathetic nerves. One characteristic feature of the renal blood flow is its autoregulation.

148. D

Sympathetic stimulation causes relaxation of the ciliary muscle for vision, relaxes the bronchiole muscle, usually decreases motility and tone in the gastrointestinal tract and causes relaxation of the detrusor muscle. It also causes constriction of the blood vessels of skin and muscle.

149. Cerbrospinal fluid

   A   has essentially the same composition as the extracellular fluid
      of the brain
   B   absorption is independent of intraventricular pressure
   C   is absorbed through the foramina of Magendie and Luschka
   D   circulates in the cerebral ventricles and subarachnoid
      plexus
   E   pressure is reduced when there is a block to cerebrospinal
      flow

150. At a synapse

   A   activity can be passed on by flow of current or release of
      a neurotransmitter
   B   chemical transmitters must be destroyed by the post
      synaptic cell
   C   there is delay in transmission of at least 0.5 msec
   D   there is 1-1 transmission
   E   nerve impulses travel in one direction only

151. Smooth muscle cells

   A   have no cross striations
   B   have no actin and myosin
   C   show spontaneous contractions
   D   have cells which are electrically coupled
   E   have conscious and autonomic control

152. Cerebellar lesions usually produce

   A   increased muscle tone
   B   resting tremor
   C   exaggerated stretch reflexes
   D   adiadokokinesia
   E   slurred or scanning speech

Answers overleaf

Physiology

149. A D

The cerebrospinal fluid has essentially the same composition as the extracellular fluid and is produced by the choroid plexus, but not purely by a process of filtration. Once formed, the fluid flows through the ventricles and finally passes out to the external surface of the central nervous system. It is absorbed through the arachnoid villi, a process which takes place largely by bulk flow and is proportional to the pressure. As cerebrospinal fluid is being formed continuously, obstruction of this circulation causes a rise in hydrostatic pressure.

150. A C E

Chemical transmission occurs at most synapses, but electrical transmission does occur. Acetyl choline, a commonly occuring transmitter, is removed by presynaptic terminals or destroyed by cholinesterase produced by cholinergic nerve terminals. Active re-uptake is important in the removal of noradrenaline. Transmission occurs in one direction only with a delay. Cells at synapses derive inputs from large numbers of axons.

151. A C D

Smooth muscle cells have no cross striations, but do possess actin and myosin. Single unit smooth muscle can contract spontaneously and action potentials may be conducted from cell to cell allowing large numbers of cells to contract spontaneously. In addition to spontaneous contraction, activity may also arise through stimulation of the autonomic nervous system.

152. D E

Cerebellar lesions usually produce hypotonia and intention tremor. Stretch reflexes are usually inhibited. There is also slurred or scanning speech and adiadokokinesia, the inability to perform rapidly alternating opposite movement.

153. The Golgi tendon organ

A is stimulated by passive stretching of the muscle
B is stimulated by active muscle contraction
C is the receptor for the inverse stretch reflex
D transmits impulses via non-myelinated fibres
E connects with motor neurones supplying muscle antagonists

154. For the process of hearing

A axons of the acoustic nerve have their cell bodies in the
   organ of Corti
B the range of frequencies audible to man is 10-1,000 Hz
C the primary auditory cortex is located in the parietal lobe
D the tympanic membrane stops vibrating when the sound
   wave stops
E a loud sound causes reflex contraction of the tensor
   tympani stapedius

155. Parkinson's disease

A is due to a lesion in the internal capsule
B could result from phenothiazine therapy
C is treated with methyldopa
D is characterised by reduced muscle tone
E is usually associated with muscle weakness

156. Hetronymous hemianopia is commonly caused by a lesion of the

A optic tract
B optic nerve
C occiptal lobe
D tectal region of the midbrain
E optic chiasma

Answers overleaf

153. A B C E

The Golgi tendon organ supplies information about muscle tension. When the muscle is put under strain, the nerve endings of the Golgi tendon are stimulated and so respond to passive stretching or active muscle contraction. They are supplied with group 1b sensory fibres which are myelinated. The Golgi tendon also mediates a protective reflex, the inverse stretch reflex. If a very heavy load is applied to the muscle, the stretch reflex can be overridden.

154. A D E

The organ of Corti consists of sensory receptor cells transforming sound energy into action potentials, the usual range of sensitivity of the ear being 20-20,000 Hz. The primary auditory cortex is located in the temporal lobe. For faithful reproduction of sound, it is important that the membrane stops vibrating almost immediately the sound stops. Reflex contraction of the tensor tympani and stapedius is a protective mechanism preventing excessive stimulation of the auditory receptors.

155. B

Parkinsonism results from a lesion of the basal ganglion, and has also been noted as a complication of treatment with the phenothiazine group of tranquilizer drugs. Parkinsonism is characterised by an increase in muscle tone, and is not associated with muscle weakness. The symptoms of some patients are relieved when the level of dopamine in the brain is raised with L-dopa. Methyldopa is an antihypertensive agent.

156. E

When the optic chiasma is affected, as for example, by pituitary tumours, visual defects occur on the opposite sides of the visual fields (heteronymous hemianopia). A lesion of the optic tract produces defects on the same side of both visual fields, those of the optic nerve lead to blindness, while lesions of the occipital lobe produce discrete quandrantic visual field defects. There is no pupillary response to light after lesions in the tectal region.

157. A skeletal or voluntary muscle

A can comprise several hundred or several thousand fibres
B comprises multinucleate cells
C contains mainly actin in the thick filaments
D contains mainly myosin in the thin filaments
E may be innervated by parasympathetic nerves

158. With regard to the sense of pain

A the sense organs are probably free nerve endings
B section of the dorsal columns has no effect on its perception
C slow pain is due to activity of the A pain fibres
D it can be stimulated by cutting the intestine with a scalpel
E lobotomy has been performed to relieve intractable pain

159. In a stretch reflex

A the sensory ending involved is the muscle spindle
B a single synapse is involved
C the sensitivity may be increased by stimulation of γ-efferents
D impulses travel by Ia (Aα) nerve fibres
E the antagonistic muscles relax

160. The neurotransmitter acetylcholine

A is released at all preganglionic neurones
B is released from neurones which innervate blood vessels in skeletal muscle
C is released from neurones supplying sweat glands
D has the same action on smooth muscle as muscarine
E requires pseudocholinesterase for its inactivation at nerve endings

157. A B

Depending on the region in the body, a skeletal muscle can comprise a few hundred or a few thousand fibres, each fibre being a multinucleate cell. Each muscle fibre contains several hundred myofibrils, which have a characteristic banded appearance depending on interdigitation of myosin containing thick filaments and actin containing thin filaments. Skeletal muscle is innervated by the somatic nervous system.

158. A E

The identity of pain receptors is uncertain, but they are probably free nerve endings. The pain fibres pass up the dorsal columns, but section may make painful stimuli more unpleasant. Slow pain is due to activity in C pain fibres. The intestines are insensitive to cutting, burning and handling. Lobotomy has been performed to relieve intractable pain.

159. A B D E

The stretch reflex is the simplest spinal reflex involving only two neurones and one synapse. The stretch receptors in the muscle spindle are stimulated and impulses pass via Ia sensory nerve fibres to the spinal cord, where they synapse with the anterior horn cells of the same muscle. Stimulation of the sensory nerves also produces relaxation of those muscles which antagonise the action of those muscles involved in the reflex.

160. A B C D

In both the sympathetic and the parasympathetic nervous system, acetylcholine is the transmitter substance released from the terminals of the preganglionic fibres. Acetylcholine is also the transmitter at neuro-effector junctions. The postganglionic neurones which innervate sweat glands and those which supply blood vessels in skeletal muscles belong anatomically to the sympathetic nervous system, but release acetylcholine. The postganglionic effects of acetylcholine can be reproduced by muscarine. Pseudocholinesterase is capable of hydrolysing acetylcholine, but is found in blood, not at nerve endings.

PATHOLOGY

GENERAL

161. The blind loop syndrome

A   is due to stasis
B   causes bacterial overgrowth
C   causes macrocytic anaemia due to folic acid deficiency
D   is commonly caused surgically
E   may cause steatorrhoea due to excessive conjugation of bile salts

162. The following conditions may cause ventilatory failure

A   chronic bronchitis
B   pulmonary emboli
C   idiopathic fibrosing alveolitis
D   pneumothorax
E   morphine

163. The following statements are true of diseases inherited as a dominant character:

A   the diseases are not usually severe enough to prevent reproduction
B   the birth of an abnormal child is usually the first indication of the condition
C   the affected members are usually heterozygous
D   haemophilia is an example of such a disease
E   affected members of the family need not usually fear transmitting the disease to their children

164. Osteoporosis

A   can be defined as a lesion in which the volume of bone tissue per unit volume of anatomical bone is reduced
B   can be caused by protein deficiency
C   when caused by prolonged immobilisation is associated with hypercalciuria
D   is seen in vitamin D deficiency
E   can be simulated radiologically by hyperparathyroidism

Answers overleaf

81

161. **A B D**

In the blind loop syndrome, stasis of enteric contents allows bacteria to proliferate. The blind loop syndrome may cause a macocytic anaemia due to B_{12} deficiency, but folate levels are normal or raised, since the organisms synthesise folate which is then absorbed. Surgery in Crohn's disease or for peptic ulcer may involve the formation of a blind loop.

162. **A D E**

Respiratory failure may be due to an inadequate volume of inspired air available for exchange (ventilatory failure), or impaired alveolar-arterial gas exchange. Pulmonary emboli and fibrosing alveolitis impair gas exchange in a normally-ventilated lung. The remainder all reduce ventilation.

163. **A C**

If a dominant gene produced a defect severe enough to prevent reproduction, it would soon disappear. B is characteristic of diseases caused by a recessive gene. Haemophilia is inherited as a sex-linked recessive character. If a gene is dominant, then unaffected members of a family need not fear transmitting the disease.

164. **A B C E**

In osteoporosis, the bone is normal in quality, but reduced in quantity. In immobilisation, the bone 'atrophies' and the net resorption causes hypercalciuria. Vitamin D deficiency causes osteomalacia, in which there is a relative lack of bone mineral compared to osteoid.

165. **Dissecting aneurysms**

    A   are the most frequent type of aortic aneurysm
    B   are due to haemorrhage occurring in the intima
    C   are confined to the upper aorta
    D   are initiated by a rupture of one of the vasa vasarum
    E   usually rupture externally

166. **The following statements are true of venous thromboembolic disease:**

    A   there may be no clinical manifestations
    B   it may be associated with hypercholesterolaemia
    C   it may cause pulmonary hypertension
    D   it may form coralline thrombus
    E   it may complicate splenectomy

167. **The following conditions caused centrizonal necrosis of the liver:**

    A   yellow fever
    B   congestive heart failure
    C   phosphorus poisoning
    D   eclampsia
    E   carbon tetrachloride

168. **In Fallot's tetralogy**

    A   there is right ventricular hypertrophy
    B   there is central cyanosis
    C   the aorta is displaced to the left
    D   there may be an associated patent ductus
    E   thrombotic complications occur

Answers overleaf

165. D E

Dissecting aneurysms are less common in the aorta than true aneurysms. They are due to haemorrhage from a vava vavorum extending into the media. They normally commence in the upper aorta, but frequently extend down the aorta.

166. A C D E

Phlebothrombosis is often asymptomatic. Repeated embolisation may lead to progressive pulmonary hypertension if the emboli are of a size insufficient to cause sudden death. Thrombosis in veins starts as a coralline thrombus which continues as a propagated clot. Splenectomy predisposes to phlebothrombosis more than most surgical operations since it induces a thrombocytosis.

167. B E

Yellow fever causes midzonal necrosis. Phosphorus poisoning and eclampsia affect the peripheral part of hepatic lobules (periportal necrosis). Congestive heart failure and carbon tetrachloride poisoning affect the central zone predominantly.

168. A B D E

In Fallot's tetralogy, there is pulmonary stenosis, (leading to) right ventricular hypertrophy, a ventricular septal defect, and overriding of the V.S.D. by the aorta. The aorta is thus displaced to the right. There may be a patent ductus. Thrombotic complications may result from the polycythaemia which arises in response to the cyanosis.

Pathology

169. Crohn's disease

A may involve the colon
B causes intestinal fistulae
C involves only mucosa and submucosa
D is often associated with hypergammaglobulinaemia
E produces crypt abcesses

170. Left ventricular failure may be due to

A mitral regurgitation
B pulmonary hypertension
C mitral stenosis
D coarctation of aorta
E aortic valve disease

171. Pulmonary infarcts

A occur in normal people if a main pulmonary artery is
   occluded
B may be complicated by a haemorrhagic pleural effusion
C are usually caused by an embolus from the leg veins
D are usually caused by primary thrombosis of the pulmonary
   arteries
E do not commonly produce haemoptysis

172. The following conditions may cause high-output cardiac failure:

A anaemia
B advanced liver disease
C amyloid disease
D cor pulmonale
E shock

169. A B D E

Crohn's disease may involve any part of the alimentary tract, from lips to anus. It causes transmural inflammation; fissures develop which may pass through the bowel wall to form fistulae. As in other chronic inflammatory diseases, there is a hyper-gammaglobulinaemia. Crypt abcesses are commonly seen in both ulcerative colitis and Crohn's disease; their presence in no way allows a distinction to be made between the 2 diseases.

170. A D E

The left ventricle fails when it is subjected to an increased work-load, as in mitral regurgitation, aortic valve disease, co-arctation of the aorta, and systemic hypertension, or when it is subjected to a reduced blood supply, as in coronary artery thrombosis. Mitral stenosis and pulmonary hypertension do not increase the work-load on the left ventricle.

171. B C

Occlusion of the pulmonary artery does not, by itself, cause infarction since bronchial arteries provide an adequate arterial supply to sustain viability. If there is also a poor cardiac output, this supply becomes insufficient. Infarction causes weakening of vessel walls through which red cells can escape into the pleural cavity (haemorrhagic pleural effusion) and into bronchi (haemoptysis). Thrombosis of pulmonary arteries is a rare cause of pulmonary infarction, occurring only in severe pulmonary hypertension.

172. A B D

Anaemia causes high-output cardiac failure when the oxygen-carrying capacity of the blood becomes insufficient to supply the needs of the myocardium. Advanced liver disease causes a hyperkinetic circulation and this may rarely lead to high-output heart failure. Amyloid embarrasses the action of the heart and may cause low output failure. Cor pulmonale may cause high-output failure to be superimposed by the hypoxic hypoxia which is often part of this condition.

173. A sudden reduction of more than 20% of the blood volume produces

A an increased blood flow to the kidneys
B an increased platelet count
C increased fibrinolysis
D a fall in arterial pH
E a lowering of body temperature

174. Emboli

A may form during an operation on the head and neck
B may originate in a pregnant uterus
C commonly cause a haemorrhage
D are a common cause of aortic aneurysms
E may form after multiple fractures

175. The following are true of gall-stones

A 'mixed' stones are usually single, large round stones
B they are found in about 75% of cases of cancer of the gall bladder
C pigment stones are an important complication of acquired haemolytic anaemias
D acute ascending cholangitis may complicate a stone in the common bile duct
E the commonest type of stone is the calcium carbonate type

176. Goitre

A can develop in iodine deficiency states
B can develop in iodine excess states
C can occur in vegetarians
D never occurs in Hashimoto's disease
E occasionally extends behind the sternum into the posterior mediastinum

Answers overleaf

Pathology

173. B C D E

There is renal vasoconstriction leading to oliguria or even anuria. There is a thrombocythaemia and a transient increase in fibrinolysis. Haemorrhage causes a metabolic acidosis. Body temperature falls due to decreased heat production.

174. A B E

Low venous pressure in the upper part of the body predisposes to the entry of air into open veins, causing air embolus. Rupture of uterine veins may allow amniotic fluid to enter the venous circulation. Fractures may cause globules of fat to enter the venous circulation.

175. B D

Almost all stones are mixed; stones are usually multiple and faceted. Stones are usually present in gallbladders containing a carcinoma. Pigment stones commonly complicate congenital haemolytic anaemias, but not acquired ones. The stagnation of bile following ductal obstruction predisposes to acute cholongitis if in the common duct. Calcium carbonate stones are rare.

176. A B C

Goitre develops when the thyroid increases in size to compensate for reduced iodine intake. Iodine excess can interfere with organic iodide transport and metabolism, causing hypothyroidism and compensatory goitre formation. Some vegetables, particularly cabbage, contain substances which interfere with thyroid hormone formation (goitrogens). Hashimoto's disease commonly causes a firm goitre. Goitre may extend into the mediastinum, but always into the superior or anterior parts.

177. Manifestations of hepatic failure are

A the plasma volume is decreased due to pooling in the splanchnic area
B flapping tremor and palmar erythema
C bleeding tendencies due to failure of synthesis of clotting factors including factors VII and VIII
D breast atrophy in women
E ascites which is associated with hypoalbuminaemia and hyperaldosteronism

178. Increased skin pigmentation may be found in

A haemosiderosis
B myxoedema
C pellagra
D Cushing's syndrome
E pregnancy

179. Which of the following may cause portal hypertension?

A schistosomiasis
B congestive splenomegaly
C hepatic vein thrombosis
D oesophageal varices
E hepatic cirrhosis

180. The following may result in the formation of bone cysts:

A hyperparathyroidism
B giant cell tumour of bone
C multiple myeloma
D pulmonary osteoarthropathy
E ependymoma

Answers overleaf

177. B D E

The plasma volume is increased in hepatic failure mainly due to salt retention (due to hyperaldosteronism). There is flapping tremor, a manifestation of hepatic enuphalopathy, and palmar erythema (of unknown aetiology, but possibly due eostrogen excess). There are bleeding tendencies due to reduced clotting factor synthesis, but factor VIII is not produced by the liver. Women develop amenorrhoea and breast atrophy (men may develop gynaecomastia and testicular atrophy). Ascites is common in hepatic failure, due to a combination of hypoalbuminaemia and hyperaldosteronism.

178. C E

In haemosiderosis, the excess iron is stored in cells of the liver, pancreas, heart and the reticuloendothelial system. There is no increased skin pigmentation. Haemochromatosis causes increased skin pigmentation. Increased skin pigmentation may be seen in thyrotoxicosis, but is not seen in myxoedema. Pellagra, caused by niacin deficiency, causes a chronic erythema and dermatitis. Cushing's syndrome is caused by excess glucocorticoids; Addison's disease, due to deficient glucocorticoid production, causes hyperpigmentation via stimulation of ACTH production (and possibly MSH). If hyperpigmentation develops in a patient with Cushing's syndrome, it is called Nelson's syndrome (again due to ACTH/MSH excess). Hyperpigmentation is sometimes seen in pregnancy, mainly over the nipples, genitalia and face.

179. A C E

Schistosomiasis causes fibrosis around portal tracts (presinusoidal portal hypertension). Congestive splenomegaly and oesophageal varices are caused by portal hypertension. Hepatic vein thrombosis causes a post-sinusoidal portal hypertension.

180. A B

Hyperparathyroidism can cause sufficient bone resorption to cause bone cysts (osteitis fibrosa cystica). Giant cell tumours of bone erode the mineralised tissue to cause cystic radiolucencies. Although multiple myeloma causes radiolucenies, these are not cystic, but consist of masses of plasma cells. Pulmonary osteoarthropathy leads to increased bone density (sub-periosteal new bone formation) around wrists and ankles. Ependymomas are tumours arising in the ventricles of the brain and the central canal of the spinal cord.

181. Amyloidosis

    A is characterised by the presence of extracellular basophilic hyaline material
    B may be demonstrated by congo red dye which stains the amyloid orange
    C is deposited perireticularly in the spleen
    D is often found extensively in medullary carcinoma of the thyroid
    E may be a complication of Hodgkin's disease

182. The following changes may occur in cirrhosis of the liver:

    A retention of salt and water
    B depressed serum cholesterol
    C depressed level of serum factor VIII
    D pyrexia
    E elevated serum vitamin B_{12}

INFLAMMATION AND REPAIR

183. Benign chronic gastric ulcer

    A has a high risk of malignant change
    B is caused by hypersecretion of gastric acid
    C is seen in the acid-producing area of mucosa
    D may produce hour-glass deformity of the stomach
    E is commoner in women

184. In the tuberculous lesion

    A there is an initial infiltration by polymorphs
    B normally there is progressive destruction of organisms by macrophages
    C caseation consists of dead polymorphs and dead tissue cells
    D the evidence of healing is the presence of numerous giant cells
    E the diagnosis can be made by the presence of caseation, macrophages and epithelioid cells

Answers overleaf

181. B C D E

Amyloid is eosinophilic. It can be demonstrated with congo red, or methyl violet. If stained with congo red, it shows a green birefringence in polarised light. It is deposited around reticulin fibres in various organs, and in blood vessels. In medullary carcinoma of the thyroid, amyloid is extensively deposited around the tumour cells, and represents a degradation product of their secretion. Amyloid is deposited in many chronic inflammatory and malignant diseases.

182. A B D E

There is salt and water retention due to hyperaldosteronism. Cholesterol is manufactured in the liver and falls in cirrhosis. Factor VIII remains normal—it is not manufactured by the liver but by vascular endothelium. A low-grade pyrexia, uninfluenced by antibiotics or diet, is not uncommon during the course of cirrhosis. Vitamin B12, stored in the liver, may rise with release from damaged liver cells: liver cell damage is a continuing feature of cirrhosis.

183. D

The incidence of carcinoma developing in a benign gastric ulcer is less than 1%. Since patients with gastric ulcer are predisposed to the development of carcinoma elsewhere in the stomach, even this low incidence may not be a casual association. The acid output in stomachs with gastric ulcer is normal or low. Carcinomas develop in areas which do not produce acid. They are commoner in men.

184. A B

There is transient acute inflammation, but polymorphs soon become replaced by mononuclear cells. Macrophages normally progressively destroy the organisms, and this killing capacity is largely dependent upon the immune system. Caseous tissue consists of dead macrophages and dead tissue cells. Giant cells are seen as part of the tissue response to tuberculosis, but do not infer healing. The diagnosis is made by finding the organism. Caseating granulomas are highly suggestive but not conclusive evidence of tuberculosis.

185. The outcome of acute inflammation may be

A chronic inflammation
B malignancy
C calcification
D graft versus host reaction
E resolution

186. The following are features of bronchopneumonia

A it is commonest in infancy and old age
B it is usually due to highly virulent pneumococcus
C it usually affects only one lung
D it can be produced by a foreign body obstructing a
    bronchus
E it usually affects previously healthy people

187. Amyloid disease may be a sequel to

A rheumatoid arthritis
B subacute bacterial endocarditis
C multiple sclerosis
D chronic suppurative disease
E leprosy

188. Acute inflammation

A results in a decrease in blood flow to the affected part
B produces increased vascular permeability to proteins
C is associated with local 5—hydroxytryptamine release
D may be caused by mechanical trauma
E is the manifestation of the ability of normal tissues to
    respond to damage

Answers overleaf

185. A C E

Chronic inflammation commonly follows acute inflammation if the inflammatory agent persists. There is no evidence to suggest that acute inflammation predisposes to malignancy. Calcification may occur in the walls of abcess cavities. When there is relatively little tissue damage, the acute inflammation may resolve without permanent tissue changes. A good example is lobar pneumonia.

186. A D

Bronchopneumonia usually affects people of low resistance, and is most common at the extremes of life. It is usually caused by organisms of relatively low virulence, unlike lobar pneumonia which is caused by the highly virulent pneumococcus. It is nearly always bilateral, unless it is produced by the stasis imposed by an obstructive lesion.

187. A D E

The common type of amyloid disease, secondary amyloidosis, is seen as a sequel to chronic inflammatory diseases. In the past, it was a common sequel to pulmonary tuberculosis, osteomyelitis, bronchiectosis and tertiory syphilis. Nowadays, it is more commonly the sequel to rheumatoid arthritis, leprosy, inflammatory bowel disease and certain malignant diseases, especially Hodgkin's disease.

188. B C D E

Acute inflammation is associated with an increased vascular perfusion. The capillaries become more permeable. 5—hydroxytryptamine release is an early event in acute inflammation. Acute inflammation is the local response of tissues to injury, which includes mechanical injury; the tissue must remain alive to be able to participate in the inflammatory response.

189. Chronic pyelonephritis

  A is often associated with infection by gram negative cocci
  B may commence either as an overt acute disease or may appear insidiously
  C is the commonest cause of chronic renal failure
  D affects the glomeruli
  E does not cause hypertension

190. The following are associated with a giant cell reaction:

  A traumatic fat necrosis
  B fungal infections
  C tuberculosis
  D syphilis
  E systemic amyloidosis

191. The metabolic response to injury includes

  A increased secretion of ADH
  B elevation of serum growth hormone
  C increased urinary excretion of potassium
  D increased secretion of renin
  E impaired glucose tolerance

192. The following factors may adversely affect the healing of wounds:

  A exposure to ionising radiation
  B exposure to ultraviolet light
  C vitamin C deficiency
  D low temperatures
  E direction of the skin wound

Answers overleaf

189. B C D

Chronic pyelonephritis is associated with infection by gram negative intestinal bacilli. Although the disease is predominantly one of tubules and pelvis, when a tubule is destroyed, its supplying glomerulus becomes hyalinised. Chronic pyelonephritis causes hypertension.

190. A B C D

Inflammatory giant cells are seen in tissues in association with the presence of many substances, whether of endogenous origin (e.g. bile, lipids escaped from cells, keratin) or exogenous (sutures, mycobacteria). Giant cells are seen around syphilitic gummas, although not so conspicuously as in tuberculosis. They are not a feature of amyloidosis, although they are sometimes seen around certain types of localised amyloid (e.g. that seen in medullary carcinoma of thyroid).

191. A B C D E

Increased secretion of ADH, which conserves water by increasing reabsorption in the renal tubules, is caused by increased osmolarity of hypothalamic extracellular fluid (osmoreceptors), reduced blood volume (via baroreceptors), and is also caused by pain, fear, nicotine etc. Growth hormone levels rise in stress, as do glucocorticoids, which impair glucose tolerance. Stress also stimulates renin secretion, which serves to conserve sodium (via angiotension) at the expense of increased potassium loss.

192. A C D E

Ionising radiation damages tissue during exposure and causes a permanently reduced vascularity in exposed tissues, and this reduced vascularity impairs healing. Ultraviolet light has been shown clinically and experimentally to promote wound healing. Vitamin C deficiency impairs wound healing (vitamin C is needed in collagen metabolism). Wounds heal more slowly in cold tissues, and the rate of wound healing is directly proportional to the tissue temperature. Wounds heal much faster if the skin incision is parallel to the lines of Langer.

TUMOURS

193. **The following are true of testicular teratomas:**

A   they are usually predominantly cystic
B   most of them are benign
C   they usually occur in young and middle-aged men
D   they sometimes produce chorionic gonadotrophins giving rise to a positive pregnancy test
E   they are slow to metastasize

194. **Squamous metaplasia occurs in the following:**

A   colon
B   renal pelvis
C   uterus
D   alveoli
E   prostate

195. **Oat cell carcinoma of the bronchus**

A   is the commonest form of bronchial neoplasm
B   is radiosensitive
C   is more common in women than in men
D   is composed of eosinophilic cells
E   is a recognised site of ectopic ACTH secretion

196. **Osteogenic sarcoma**

A   occurs most commonly in late childhood
B   the cell of origin is the osteoclast
C   often has numerous giant cells
D   is confined by epiphyseal cartilage
E   spreads early via the lymphatics

Answers overleaf

193. C D

The testicular teratoma is very different from the common type of ovarian teratoma ('dermoid cyst'). It is a predominantly solid tumour, although it may show small cystic spaces. They are almost always malignant, and metastasize rapidly by blood and lymphatics. They occur in young and middle-aged men. They may produce chorionic gonadotrophins, responsible for a positive pregnancy test.

194. B E

Epithelial metaplasia is a condition in which there is a change of one type of differentiated epithelium to another type of epithelial tissue. Squamous metaplasia can occur in the gall bladder, renal pelvis, urinary bladder, uterus, bronchi and prostate gland.

195. B E

The commonest tumour of the bronchus is a squamous cell carcinoma. Oat cell carcinomas compose about 20% of primary lung carcinomas (squamous 40%). The oat cell carcinoma is radiosensitive, and composed of small basophilic cells with round or oval nuclei. They are associated with smoking and are more common in men than women. They are thought to be derived from neurosecretory cells in the bronchus, and are a recognised site of ectopic hormone production.

196. A C D

Osteogenic sarcomas are commonest in late childhood, with a second minor incidence hump in old age (due to Paget's disease). They are tumours of osteoblasts, although there may be numerous osteoclastic giant cells amongst the tumour cells. Epiphyseal cartilage has a delaying effect on tumour spread. Spread is characteristically by the blood stream.

197. The following are characteristic features of malignant tumours:

A   abnormal mitoses
B   anaplasia
C   reactive hyperplasia in regional nodes
D   increased fibrous stroma
E   invasiveness

198. The following are characteristic features of Hodgkin's disease:

A   it commonly presents with an intermittent pyrexia of
    unknown origin
B   reticulum cells show a large number of mitotic figures
C   if associated with few lymphocytes indicates a
    favourable prognosis
D   if limited to a single node group has a 40% 15-year
    survival rate with radiotherapy
E   the lymph nodes are soft and have a white appearance when
    cut across

199. The carcinoid syndrome

A   may produce tricuspid incompetence
B   may produce bronchospasm
C   often results from a carcinoid of rectum
D   suggests liver metastases if the tumour is of
    gastro-intestinal origin
E   may be due to a bronchial adenoma

200. The following conditions are premalignant

A   keratoacanthoma
B   cystic hyperplasia of the breast
C   leukoplakia
D   senile keratosis
E   intestinal polyposis coli

Answers overleaf

197. A B E

Malignant tumours generally show an increased number of mitotic figures, amongst which some are abnormal. Anaplasia is a term used to denote lack of resemblance of the malignant tumour tissue to its parent tissue. Although regional nodes often do show reactive hyperplasia, this effect may follow many other causes, and cannot be said to be characteristic of malignant tumours. The amount of fibrous stroma present in a tumour varies enormously: some have much (e.g. scirrhous carcinoma of breast), some have very little (e.g. encephaloid tumours of breast). All malignant tumours are invasive.

198. B D

There is usually little in the way of constitutional symptoms at presentation, which is commonly as lymphadenopathy. Reticulum cells are felt to be the neoplastic element of the lymph node enlargement, and many mitoses can usually be found amongst them. When binucleate they are termed 'Reed-Sternberg' cells. The presence of large numbers of lymphocytes confers a favourable prognosis. Cases which are treated adequately when only a single node group is involved can effectively be cured. Lymph nodes are characteristically pink and firm.

199. A B D E

The carcinoid syndrome is associated with bronchospasm, and sometimes pulmonary vascular reflexes cause a functional tricuspid incompetence. Structural tricuspid incompetence can also develop due to valvular thickenings. Rectal carcinoids do not cause the carcinoid syndrome. A very high proportion of gastro-intestinal carcinoids which produce the carcinoid syndrome have metastasised: the hormonal mediators of the carcinoid syndrome are inactivated in the liver. Bronchial adenomas can produce the carcinoid syndrome (in this instance the valvular lesions are L-sided.)

200. C D E

Although keratoacanthoma contains cells which resemble those of a squamous carcinoma, and can lead to a difficult differential diagnosis for the histopathologist, the lesion is not a premalignant condition. Cystic hyperplasia is not generally regarded as a premalignant condition, since the lesions do not commonly progress to malignancy (although there is a definite association between cystic hyperplasia and carcinoma).

201. The following statement(s) is/are true of multiple myeloma:

   A it may cause hypocalcaemia
   B the abnormal protein is usually of a heterogenous nature
   C it is usually diagnosed by the increased number of plasma cells in the peripheral blood
   D is characterised by extraskeletal lesions
   E is a tumour of plasma cells

202. The growth of the following neoplasms is often hormonally dependent:

   A prostatic carcinoma
   B follicular carcinoma of the thyroid
   C atrial myxosarcoma
   D rhabdomyosarcoma
   E oat cell carcinoma

203. The following statement(s) is/are true of malignant metastases:

   A the commonest organ in which blood-borne metastases occur is the liver
   B of the lung tumours, oat cell carcinoma is particularly liable to metastasise to the skeleton
   C osseous metastases are commonly osteosclerotic
   D multiple cutaneous deposits are characteristic of malignant melonoma
   E of the endocrine glands, the thyroid is most frequently the site of metastases

204. Inhaled asbestos

   A increases the incidence of carcinoma of the lung
   B is picked up by macrophages
   C produces diffuse fibrosis in the lungs
   D is associated with an increased incidence of pulmonary tuberculosis
   E is seen in sputum as dumb-bell shaped bodies

Answers overleaf

201. E

Multiple myeloma causes hypercalcaemia due to demineralisation of the skeleton. The protein produced is the immunoglobulin (whole or part) produced by the progeny of one cell (a clone), therefore monoclonal. Plasma cells are not generally seen in the peripheral blood—they may be found in a bone marrow aspirate. Extraskeletal tumours are rare (plasmacytomas).

202. A B

Stilboestrol frequently causes at least temporary and partial regression of prostatic carcinomas. Follicular carcinoma of the thyroid frequently responds to thyroid hormone administration, although this is not the treatment of choice. Oat cell carcinomas may produce one or more hormones, but are not hormonally dependent.

203. A B D

The liver is the commonest organ for blood-borne metastases, not only from gastro-intestinal but genitourinary, breast *and* lung carcinomas, and melanomas. The lung is the second commonest site. Squamous, adeno and large-cell undifferentiated carcinomas only occasionally produce skeletal metastases. Osseous metastases are almost always osteolytic, the exceptions being prostatic, and occasional breast carcinomas. Melanoma shows a prediliction for metastasis to skin. The adrenal gland is the endocrine gland most commonly the site for metastases.

204. A B C D E

All types of asbestos predispose to carcinoma of the lung, particularly in smokers, although crocidolite is more strongly associated with mesothelioma than the other types. The fibres are ingested by macrophages, or if too large, several macrophages aggregate around the material. Asbestos inhalation produces diffuse interstitial fibrosis. It predisposes to tuberculosis. Asbestos bodies are dumb-bell shaped structures of asbestos coated with iron, which is seen in the sputum of individuals who have inhaled asbestos fibres.

205. **An acidophil adenoma of the pituitary gland may produce**

   A acromegaly
   B Cushing's syndrome
   C paroxysmal hypertension
   D increased secretion of urinary catacholamines
   E osteitis fibrosa cystica

MICROBIOLOGY/IMMUNOLOGY

206. **Gas gangrene**

   A is caused by *Clostridium septicum*
   B can be caused by bacteroides
   C symptoms are caused by endotoxins
   D spreads because of hyaluranidase production by the organism
   E causes haemolytic anaemia

207. **The clinical manifestations of anaphylactic shock are due to**

   A spasm of bronchial smooth muscle
   B damage to small blood vessels and an increase in their permeability
   C sludging of red cells
   D antigen and antibody reaction
   E spasm of smooth muscle in the blood vessels

208. **Staphylococci**

   A are gram-positive spherical motile organisms
   B are arranged in chains
   C are facultative anaerobes
   D some produce an exotoxin
   E may produce coagulase

Answers overleaf

205. A

Acidophil adenomas secrete growth hormone, leading to gigantism or acromegaly. Occasionally they can secrete prolactin. Cushing's syndrome is caused by a basophil adenoma. Paroxysmal hypertension is due to to phaeochromocytomas, due to increased catecholamine secretion; osteitis fibrosa cystica is caused by parathyroid gland overactivity (hyperplasia, adenoma or carcinoma).

206. A D E

Gas gangrene is caused by infection by *Cl. welchii, Cl. septicum* and *Cl. oedematiens*. Spores germinate in anaerobic tissue, and, once established cause spreading necrosis by releasing histotoxic erotoxins. Gas is formed by anaerobic fermentation of tissue components. The infection spreads rapidly by breaking down ground substances with hyaluronidase and collagenase. Exotoxins also reach the circulation where they cause profound shock and haemolytic anaemia.

207. A B D E

The main effects of anaphylaxis are spasm of smooth muscle (bronchial and arteriolar) with damage to small blood vessels with an increase in their permeability. It is dependent on reaction between antigen and antibody, the antibody being either IgE (on mast cells) or free in the circulation, when immune complexes are formed.

208. C D E

Staphylococci are gram positive spherical organisms but they are nonmotile. They are arranged in clusters, in contradistinction to the chains formed by streptococci. They are aerobic organisms, but can tolerate an anaerobic environment. *Staphylococcus aureus* produces several exotoxins, including coagulase, hyaluronidase and staphylokinase. Some strains also produce an exotoxin called enterotoxin.

209. The following organisms are naturally pathogenic to both man and animals:

A   *Bordetella pertussis*
B   *Brucella abortus*
C   *Neisseria gonorrhoeae*
D   *Salmonella typhi*
E   *Treponema pallidum*

210. The following organisms are usually sensitive to penicillin

A   Neisseria
B   Pseudomonas
C   Pneumococcus
D   *E. coli*
E   Rickettsiae

211. Endotoxins are

A   heat labile
B   strongly antigenic
C   inactivated solely by antibody
D   liberated when the organism is destroyed
E   proteins

212. Which of the following is/are the site(s) of immunoglobulin synthesis?

A   red cells
B   platelets
C   plasma cells
D   fibroblasts
E   eosinophils

Answers overleaf

209. **B**

    Bordetella pertussis, Neisseria gonorrhoeae, Salmonella typhi and *Treponema pallidum* are pathogenic only to man.

210. **A C**

    Penicillin is the drug of choice against pneumococcus and neisseria. The gram negative bacilli generally, including pseudomonas and *E. coli*, are resistant. Tetracycline is the drug of choice against rickettsiae.

211. **D**

    Endotoxins are complexes of protein and lipopolysaccharide. They are heat-stable and generally weakly antigenic. They can interact with complement by the alternative pathway in the absence of antibody. Small amounts are liberated from living organisms, large amounts when the organisms are destroyed.

212. **C**

    Immunoglobulins are produced by plasma cells, which differentiate from small lymphocytes.

213. **Actinomycosis**

    A   most commonly occurs in the ileocaecal region
    B   spreads via the lymphatics
    C   tends to produce chronic fistulae
    D   commonly exhibits giant cells at the periphery of the lesion
    E   extends along tissue planes

214. **The long-term survival of homografts is improved by**

    A   Hodgkin's disease
    B   thymic deficiency syndromes
    C   uraemia
    D   pregnancy
    E   azathiaprine adminstration

215. **B-haemolytic streptococci**

    A   cause erysipelas
    B   cause synergistic gangrene
    C   cause puerperal sepsis
    D   produce hyaluronidase
    E   produce a cardiotoxic endotoxin

216. **A homograft**

    A   is a transplant made from one site to another in the same individual
    B   would describe a renal transplant from one person, dead or alive, to another
    C   will never undergo a second set phenomenon
    D   given as a second set may have its survival time prolonged if the host undergoes irradiation
    E   may survive longer when transplanted into the brain

Answers overleaf

213. C

65% of cases of actinomycosis infection are cervicofacial. The organism does not involve the lymphatics, but spreads by direct invasion and the blood stream. The infection is characterised by granulamatous inflammation. Pus cells surround the colonies, and around these inflammatory granulation tissue and fibrosis develop. Giant cells are not a feature.

214. A B C D E

Hodgkin's disease, thymic deficiency syndromes and uraemia all impair the immune response and hence prolong homograft survival. Graft rejection is also reduced in pregnancy, and by **azathiaprine** administration.

215. B C D E

B-haemolytic streptococci *(Streptococcus pyogenes)* cause erysepelas. They produce many exotoxins, including hyaluranidase, and toxic products which are intermediate between endotoxins and exotoxins including streptolysin O, which is cardiotoxic.

216. B E

A homograft is a transplant made from one individual to another of the same species. A graft from one site to another on the same individual is an autograft. The second set phenomemon is the rapid rejection by the recipient of a second homograft from the same donor. Although whole-body irradiation prolongs the life of a primary homograft, it does not affect survival time of second set grafts. Some special sites allow prolonged graft survival. The best example is the anterior chamber of the eye, but the brain also allows prolonged survival.

HAEMATOLOGY

217. Haemolytic transfusion reactions commonly occur

A   when transfusing blood with a high titre of plasma
    agglutinins against recipient cells
B   when transfusing blood into patients with high plasma
    titres of agglutinins against donor red cells
C   when transfusing blood type A into subjects of blood group
    AB
D   when transfusing blood of type O into subjects of blood
    group A
E   when transfusing rhesus negative blood into rhesus
    positive recipients.

218. A prolonged prothrombin time is normally found in:

A   haemolytic jaundice
B   liver failure
C   adrenal failure
D   factor VII deficiency
E   malabsorption with steatorrhoea

219. Splenectomy may be of value in the treatment of

A   idiopathic thrombocytopenic purpura
B   heriditary spherocytosis
C   lymphocyte-depleted Hodgkin's disease
D   infectious mononucleosis
E   malaria

**220. Which of the following could be transmitted by blood
transfusions?**

A   amoebiasis
B   tuberculosis
C   malaria
D   Crohn's disease
E   hepatitis

Answers overleaf

217. B

Transfusion of agglutinins does not usually cause haemolysis, because they are diluted by recipient blood below damaging levels. Subjects of blood group AB are 'universal recipients' producing no major blood group antibodies. Subjects of group O are 'universal donors', possessing no major blood group antigens. Similarly, rhesus negative red cells do not have rhesus group antigens on their surface to allow anti-rhesus antibodies to effect haemolysis.

218. B D E

Prothrombin time is prolonged in obstructive jaundice because vitamin K, required for prothrombin production, is not absorbed in the absence of bile salts. Hepatic failure reduces hepatic synthesis of prothrombin. The prothrombin time assay measures the integrity of the extrinsic system (factor VII) and the common pathway (factor X, VII and prothrombin). Deficiency of any of these factors causes a prolonged prothrombin time. In malabsorption and steatorrhoea, vitamin K is not absorbed and therefore the prothrombin time is prolonged.

219. A B C D

The spleen is the major effector of the increased destruction of platelets in thrombocytopenic purpura, and of red cells in hereditary spherocytosis; its removal may reduce the rate of destruction. Splenectomy is often performed in Hodgkin's disease, and has value both in removing involved tissue if the spleen is involved, and in staging the disease to allow appropriate therapeutic decisions to be made. Splenectomy may become essential in infectious mononucleosis if the spleen ruptures.

220. C E

Amoebae are not present in blood, transmission is feco-oral. Tuberculosis may be transmitted by inhalation, ingestion or inoculation. Malaria is a blood parasite and can be thus transmitted. Several forms of hepatitis can be transmitted by blood.

221. The prothrombin time may be prolonged

A   in haemophilia
B   after extra-corporeal circulation
C   in biliary obstruction
D   during heparin therapy
E   in Von Willebrand's disease

222. Which of the following may cause polycythaemia:

A   poliomyelitis
B   encephalitis
C   diabetes mellitus
D   hypernephroma
E   cyanotic congenital heart disease

223. The following changes occur after a splenectomy:

A   Howell-Jolly bodies appear in the blood and persist
indefinitely
B   there is a very transient leucocytosis
C   there is a thrombocytosis
D   in hereditary spherocytosis, the spherocytes disappear from
the blood
E   siderocytes appear in the blood

224. The following findings suggest a diagnosis of haemolytic anaemia:

A   increased reticulocytes in the peripheral blood
B   raised serum bilirubin
C   bone marrow showing normoblastic hyperplasia
D   increased iron binding capacity
E   histamine-fast achlorhydria

221. B C D

The prothrombin time is normal in haemophilia.
Extra-corporeal circulation may cause consumption of clotting factors and platelets. Biliary obstruction causes hypoprothrombinaemia due to failure to absorb vitamin K. The prothrombin time may be normal or prolonged by heparin therapy. The prothrombin time is normal in Von Willebrand's disease.

222. D E

Polycythaemia is caused by hypoxia due to chronic pulmonary disease, cyanotic heart disease and living at high altitudes. It can also occur in hypernephroma. Although Cushing's disease can cause diabetes mellitus, diabetes does not cause polycythaemia.

223. A C E

Red cell inclusions such as Howell-Jolly bodies and siderotic granules are normally removed in the spleen. There is an early nentrophil leucocytosis and a permanent rise in both lymphocytes and monocytes. There is a thrombocytosis which returns to normal after a few weeks. If splenectomy is performed for hereditary spherocytosis, the spherocytes are no longer destroyed and thus persist in the blood.

224. A B C

Increased reticulocytes in the blood represents the release of immature red cells into the blood to compensate for increased red cell loss. The elevated bilirubin is due to increased breakdown of red cells. The bone marrow compensates for the loss by increased formation, seen as normoblastic hyperplasia. An increased iron binding capacity denotes iron deficiency, not seen in haemolytic anaemia. Histamine-fast achlorhydria is seen in pernicious anaemia.

CHEMICAL

225. **The following changes are usually found in chronic renal failure:**

    A hypokalaemia
    B metabolic acidosis
    C sodium retention
    D hypercalcaemia
    E normocytic normochromic anaemia

226. **A patient with hyperparathyroidism may present with**

    A calcification of the basal ganglia
    B peptic ulceration
    C pathological fractures
    D recurrent renal calculus formation
    E oliguria

227. **In persistent vomiting due to pyloric stenosis the following may occur:**

    A oliguria
    B a low plasma bicarbonate
    C marked potassium depletion
    D an acid urine
    E a low plasma sodium

228. **In hypermagnesaemia, the following occur:**

    A peripheral vasoconstriction
    B muscular rigidity
    C drowsiness
    D hypertension
    E convulsions

Answers overleaf

Pathology

225. B C E

In chronic renal failure, there is usually a mild retention of potassium which may become severe terminally. There is a metabolic acidosis due to loss of ability to produce an acid urine. Sodium is normally excreted by kidneys and reduced renal reserve reduces sodium excretion. Kidneys normally excrete phosphate, and as phosphate excretion falls, serum phosphate rises, thus reducing the serum calcium. There is in addition, impaired vitamin D metabolism by the kidney. A normocytic normochromic anaemia usually accompanies chronic renal failure.

226. B C D

Calcification of the basal ganglia may be seen in hypoparathyroidism. Peptic ulceration may be seen in hypercalcaemia of any cause, and is thought to be due to the increased secretion of gastrin caused by hypercalcaemia. Increased bone resorption predisposes to pathological fractures. Renal calculus formation is a well-known mode of presentation. Hyperparathyroidism causes polyuria because hypercalcaemia causes the renal tubules to become unresponsive to ADH.

227. A C D E

The loss of sodium, chloride and water leads to dehydration and oliguria. Loss of hydrogen ions from the stomach raises the plasma bicarbonate. There is potassium depletion, partly through loss of gastric contents, partly due to renal conservation of sodium at the expense of potassium and hydrogen ions. This renal conservation of sodium also causes a loss of hydrogen ions into the urine, causing an acid urine to be formed despite a metabolic alkalosis. Low plasma sodium follows loss of sodium from the stomach.

228. C

Magnesium excess may be seen in chronic renal failure. There is drowsiness and even coma, with peripheral vasodilation, hypotension and muscular flaccidity. Magnesium deficiency, which is very rare, can cause convulsions.

114

229. Elevated urinary conjugated bilirubin is found in

A chlorpromazine-induced jaundice
B Dubin-Johnson syndrome
C thalassaemia
D paroxysmal nocturnal haemoglobinuria
E primary biliary cirrhosis

230. Metastatic calcification may be caused by

A carcinoma of the parathyroid gland
B hypoparathyroidism
C tertiary hyperparathyroidism
D sarcoidosis
E hypovitaminosis D

231. ACTH

A stimulates gastric acid secretion
B levels in serum show a diurnal rhythm
C levels are low in Addison's disease
D secretion is regulated by circulating
   glucocorticoid levels
E acts on the zona glumerulosa of the adrenal cortex

232. In pure water deficiency state

A the plasma sodium concentration rises
B the plasma protein concentration rises
C the packed cell volume (haematocrit) rises
D the haemoglobin concentration rises
E the urea concentration rises

Answers overleaf

229. A B E

Chlorpromazine can cause an obstructive jaundice, in turn obstructing the passage of conjugated bilirubin to the intestines, but causing its appearance in the urine. In the Dubin-Johnson syndrome there is a failure of transport of conjugated bilirubin from hepatocytes into bile canaliculi. In thalassaemia and paroxysmal nocturnal haemoglobinaemia, the haemolytic components of the diseases lead to increased unconjugated circulating bilirubin. In primary biliary cirrhosis there is a major element of obstructive jaundice.

230. A B C D

Parathyroid carcinoma is a rare cause of hypercalcaemia more commonly due to hyperplasia or adenoma, and hypercalcaemia is an important cause of metastatic calcification. Metastatic calcification can also occur, however, in hypoparathyroidism, probably due to the raised phosphate. Some cases of parathyroid hyperplasia become autonomous, and consequently serum calcium rises. Sarcoidosis can cause hypercalcaemia. Hypovitaminosis D is a cause of hypocalcaemia.

231. A B D

ACTH stimulates gastric acid secretion by stimulating glucocorticoid secretion, which itself causes increased gastric acid secretion. ACTH stimulates glucocorticoid secretion by the zona fasciculata and reticulosa; aldosterone is produced in the zona glomerulosa. ACTH levels are raised in Addison's disease (chronic adrenal insufficiency).

232. A B E

When there is a deprivation or loss of water without an accompanying depletion of electrolytes, volume receptors cause aldosterone secretion, leading to reduced sodium excretion and increased plasma sodium concentrations. Relative water lack also causes a corresponding rise in plasma protein concentration. Packed cell volume does not change, however, because red cells are also dehydrated. Plasma urea rises due to increased urea reabsorption, not through renal failure.

233. **The following disturbances may occur in uretero-colic anastamosis:**

    A   hypokalaemia
    B   metabolic alkalosis
    C   hyperchloraemic acidosis
    D   increased production of ammonia
    E   progressive pyelonephritis

234. **In obstructive jaundice**

    A   increased urinary excretion of urobilinogen occurs
    B   slight elevation of alkaline phosphatase is typical
    C   liver biopsy should be performed if liver function tests
        are typical
    D   the faeces become bulky and pale
    E   Courvoisier's law states that a palpable gallbladder
        strongly suggests stones

235. **Hyperkalaemia may be caused by**

    A   pyloric stenosis
    B   chronic diarrhoea
    C   villous adenoma of rectum
    D   Conn's syndrome
    E   Addison's disease

236. **Which of the following are manifestations of
     hepatocellular failure?**

    A   gynaecomastia
    B   polycythaemia
    C   hypoalbuminaemia
    D   decreased excretion of bromsulphalein
    E   increased sensitivity to morphine

Answers overleaf

233. A C D E

Following ureterocolic anastomasis, there is absorption of chloride and sodium from the colon and secretion of bicarbonate and potassium. There is thus a tendency for potassium depletion, and a metabolic acidosis with hyperchloraemia. Colonic organisms split urea into ammonia. The kidneys adjust their function to counteract the metabolic effects of uretero-colic anastomasis, but there is always the danger of pyelonephritis from colonic organisms ascending the ureters.

234. D

Urobilinogen is absent in obstructive jaundice. The alkaline phosphatase is usually very high. Liver biopsy is dangerous if the biliary pressure is raised. The stools become pale due to a reduced amount of bile in the faeces, and bulky due to impaired absorption of fat, due to lack of bile salts. Courvoisier's law states that a palpable gall bladder in obstructive jaundice suggests tumour.

235. E

In pyloric stenosis, there is potassium depletion due to vomiting potassium-rich gastric juice and also due to renal compensatory mechanisms which increase renal potassium loss. Villous adenomas can cause potassium loss. In Conn's syndrome (primary hyperaldosteronism) sodium is conserved by the kidney at the expense of potassium. In Addison's disease, there is hyperkalaemia and hyponatraemia.

236. A C D E

Gynaecomastia is caused by oestrogen excess, and oestrogen is normally inactivated by liver cells. Bromsulphalein excretion is a sensitive test of liver cell function. The liver normally inactivates morphine. Albumin is manufactured by the liver.

237. **Respiratory alkalosis may occur**

A during anaesthesia
B in salicylate poisoning
C in persistent vomiting
D in diabetic coma
E during hysteria

238. **Proteinuria is a feature of**

A mercury poisoning
B hypernephroma
C cirrhosis
D Cushing's syndrome
E nephrotic syndrome

239. **In primary hyperaldosteronism**

A plasma renin levels are raised
B the cause is usually due to adenoma of the zona fasciculata
C patients may present with symptoms of hypokalaemia
D is associated with a mild acidosis
E hypertension usually responds to spironolactone

240. **Acute renal failure is characterised by**

A hypertension
B hyperkalaemia
C metabolic acidosis
D dehydration
E hypercalcaemia

Answers overleaf

237. A B E

Respiratory alkalosis may be caused during anaesthesia when muscle relaxants are used and artificial ventilation is excessive. Salicylates stimulate the respiratory centre, causing overventilation. Persistent vomiting causes a metabolic alkalosis; diabetic coma a metabolic acidosis. In hysteria, the patient sometimes hyperventilates.

238. A E

Mercurial preparations such as teething powders and diuretics can cause the nephrotic syndrome, in which there is massive proteinuria. Adenocarcinoma of the kidney (hypernephroma), cirrhosis and Cushing's syndrome do not cause proteinuria. In cirrhosis, there is hypoalbuminaemia due to reduced production of albumin by the liver.

239. C E

Plasma renin is increased in secondary, decreased in primary hyperaldosteronism. Primary hyperaldosteronism results from inappropriately raised secretion of aldosterone by the cells of the zona glomerulosa (Conn's syndrome). This is usually due to an adenoma, but sometimes there is bilateral hyperplasia. Increased aldosterone secretion causes raised sodium reabsorption with increased potassium loss. There is a metabolic alkalosis as some sodium is also exchanged for hydrogen ions in the kidney. Conn's syndrome causes hypertension which usually responds to spirinolactone.

240. B C

Hypertension is found in chronic renal failure. There is a hyperkalaemia and metabolic acidosis, since normal renal function is to excrete the ingested excess of K + and H + ions. The oliguria of acute renal failure may lead to overhydration; only during recovery, in the diuretic phase, do problems of excess water and potassium loss arise. The serum calcium usually falls due to the accumulation of phosphate, itself normally excreted by the kidney.

PRACTICE EXAM

60 Questions — time allowed 2½ hours

1. The ischiorectal fossa

A   contains the pudendal canal
B   is limited medially by the rectal wall
C   is bounded laterally by the ischium directly
D   is roofed by the skin of the anal triangle
E   extends deep to the perineal membrane in the urogenital triangle

2. In the face

A   the skin gets its entire sensory supply from branches of the trigeminal nerve (V)
B   the upper lip is supplied by the ophthalmic division of V
C   the frontalis muscle is supplied by the facial nerve (VII)
D   the 'motor' supply of the skin comes from T1 and T2
E   buccinator is a 'muscle of mastication' and is therefore supplied by the trigeminal nerve

3. In the foot

A   both the tibialis anterior and tibialis posterior are responsible for inversion
B   inversion of the foot is accompanied by abduction of the forefoot
C   the peronei are responsible for eversion of the foot
D   most of the full range of inversion and eversion occurs at the midtarsal joints
E   bony factors are the most important in maintaining the lateral longitudinal arch

4. Muscles which normally have double motor innervation are

A   the diaphragm
B   trapezius
C   digastric
D   adductor magnus
E   biceps femoris

5. The oesophagus

A   passes through the diaphragm at the level of the
    eighth thoracic vertebra
B   passes through the right crus of the diaphragm
C   has a three centimetre intra-abdominal portion
D   is lined in part by squamous, and in part by columnar,
    epithelium
E   is separated from the vertebral column by the right
    posterior intercostal arteries

**6. The blood supply of the pancreas is derived from the
following arteries**

A   gastroduodenal
B   splenic
C   left gastric artery
D   right gastric artery
E   superior mesenteric artery

7. The vagus nerve

A   has a left recurrent laryngeal branch which hooks
    round the subclavian artery
B   supplies fibres which form the cardiac plexi
C   is a major distributor of preganglionic parasympathetic
    fibres
D   is sensory to the trachea and lungs
E   is secretomotor to the parotid gland

8. The stellate ganglion

A   is a combination of the parasympathetic ganglion of
    T1 with the inferior cervical ganglion
B   lies on the neck of the first rib
C   if damaged may cause pupillary dilation, flushing of
    the face, and drooping of the upper eyelid
D   sends postganglionic fibres to the vertebral artery
E   sends rami communicantes to the 5th, 6th and 7th
    cervical spinal nerves

9. **The ureter**

    A   is innervated by autonomic fibres from sacral segments
    B   is of mesodermal origin
    C   is lined by ciliated epithelium
    D   is crossed by the genitofemoral nerve on the psoas
    E   is retroperitoneal

10. **The following structures are derived from the third pharyngeal pouch**

    A   the tympanic membrane
    B   the palatine tonsil
    C   the thymic bud
    D   the superior parathyroid gland
    E   the mastoid antrum

11. **In the knee joint**

    A   in full extension, medial rotation of the femur on the tibia 'locks' the joint while standing
    B   the lower end of the femur develops an ossification centre at 40 weeks of fetal life
    C   a capsular nerve supply is received from the obturator nerve
    D   extension takes place by L5, S1 nerve roots and flexion by L3, L4 nerve roots
    E   the posterior cruciate ligament passes forwards from the head of the tibia medial to the anterior cruciate ligament

12. **The axillary artery**

    A   is the continuation of the second part of the subclavian artery
    B   passes over the second digitation of serratus anterior at the outer border of the first rib
    C   gives rise to the subscapular artery in its second part
    D   is closely related to the trunks of the brachial plexus
    E   has the axillary vein on its medial border

13. **Branches from the trunks of the brachial plexus are the**

    A long thoracic nerve (Bell)
    B nerve to subclavius
    C medial cutaneous nerve of forearm
    D thoracodorsal nerve
    E suprascapular nerve

14. **The trachea**

    A commences at the upper border of C6 vertebra
    B is 15 cms long
    C is innervated by the recurrent laryngeal nerve
    D has its carina at the T4-T5 vertebral level
    E lies anterior to the oesophagus in the posterior mediastinum

15. **In the normal fetus/embryo**

    A at birth, the primary ossification centres for the ilium,
       ischium and pubis are usually fused
    B at seven weeks, there is an umbilical hernia
    C at eight weeks, the heart is beating
    D the urogenital sinus is continuous with the allantois
    E the blood travels from the placenta in the umbilical arteries

16. **The following cranial nerves are purely motor:**

    A glossopharyngeal nerve
    B cranial accessory nerve
    C hypoglossal nerve
    D throchlear nerve
    E trigeminal nerve

17. The obturator nerve

A has a root value of L3, 4, 5
B gives articular branches to the hip and knee joints
C supplies obturator internus muscle
D supplies obturator externus muscle
E supplies gracilis muscle

18. The facial nerve (VI)

A supplies sensation to those skin areas of the face derived from the maxillary processes
B supplies motor fibres to 2nd pharyngeal arch structures
C has no branches below the mandible
D supplies the muscles responsible for blinking
E carries no sensory fibres

19. The popliteal fossa

A is bounded medially by the biceps femoris muscle
B contains the origin of the saphenous nerve
C contains the lateral cutaneous nerve of the calf
D contains the genicular branch of the posterior division of the obturator nerve
E contains the popliteal vein superficial to the tibial nerve

20. The contents of the inguinal canal are

A the vas deferens
B the broad ligament in a female
C the testicular artery
D the inferior epigastric vessels
E lymphatics from the uterus

21. **Peripheral resistance**

    A is the sum of the resistance of all vessels in the vascular
       tree
    B lies largely in the capillaries
    C lies largely in the arterioles
    D falls in excerise
    E is unchanged in exercise

22. **From an ECG, one can obtain**

    A cardiac output
    B heart rate
    C force of contraction of ventricles
    D A-V conduction time
    E information as to the presence of ectopic foci of
       excitation

23. **In a control system, negative feedback**

    A is unstable
    B is the only type found in biological systems
    C restores the regulated variable to its operating point
    D prevents alteration of the regulated variable
    E increases the value of the regulated variable

24. **Sweat glands that play a role in thermoregulation**

    A produce a hypotonic solution
    B produce a secretion comprising mainly KC1
    C are innervated by the parasympathetic nervous system
    D are innervated by the sympathetic nervous system
    E have acetylcholine as the transmitter

25. The glomerular filtration rate

A is independent of falls in mean systolic blood pressure
B can be assessed by endogenous creatinine clearance
     measurements
C rises with increases in the blood urea levels
D correlates well with body surface area
E is reduced in the presence of low plasma protein
     concentrations

26. The main features of the renal juxtaglomerular apparatus are

A efferent arteriole
B afferent arteriole
C macula densa round distal convoluted tubule
D juxtaglomerular cells containing renin granules
E renal nerves

27. Glycosuria may occur

A after physical trauma
B after mental trauma
C in the presence of normal blood glucose levels
D in gross renal tubular disease
E in diabetes insipidus

28. Glucocorticoids

A decrease the circulating eosinophils
B alter resistance of the gastric mucosa to the irritant action
     of gastric secretions
C increase protein anabolism
D increase the size of the lymph nodes
E increase glucose–6–phosphatase activity

29. Lactation

  A is initiated by a post partum prolactin surge
  B requires the presence of adequate circulating growth hormone
  C is controlled by oxytocin
  D inhibits ovulation in 50% of nursing mothers
  E occurs inappropriately in the Budd-Chiari syndrome

30. The D vitamins

  A are fat soluble
  B are stored in the liver
  C comprise two main forms: D_2 and D_3
  D if deficient result in osteomalacia in adults
  E if present in excess cause hypercalcaemia and generalised metastatic calcification

31. Prostaglandins

  A are small molecular weight polypeptides
  B are chemically related to thromboxanes
  C have been clearly shown to be responsible for luteolysis in women
  D inhibit secretion of renin
  E are produced in the seminal vesicles in man

32. In the colon

  A water is absorbed
  B sodium is secreted
  C bicarbonate is secreted
  D potassium is absorbed
  E a number of vitamins are synthesised and reabsorbed

33. **The lower small intestine is the primary site of absorption of**

  A fatty acids
  B bile salts
  C calcium
  D iron
  E vitamin B_{12}

34. **Intracranial pressure may be increased by**

  A an increase in venous pressure
  B hypocapnia
  C hypoxia
  D hypothermia
  E negative g (acceleration downward, force acting towards the head)

35. **Following the passage of an action potential, there is a period of hyperpolarisation**

  A when the nerve cell is more excitable than at rest
  B when the membrane potential is 10-20mV less than at rest
  C produced by a sudden massive influx of sodium
  D which is influenced by agents that inhibit metabolism
  E which lasts for 35-40 msec

36. **The blood brain barrier**

  A is poorly developed at birth
  B is not present in the posterior pituitary
  C is not broken by tumours
  D can be easily crossed by dopamine
  E can be easily crossed by penicilline

37. **The muscle spindle**

    A   supplies the central nervous system with information
           concerning muscle length
    B   supplies the central nervous system with information
           concerning muscle tension
    C   is sensitized by fusimotor nerve activity
    D   possesses two types of sensory ending
    E   contributes to the tone of the surrounding muscle

38. **Given the following data:**

    pH 7.31
    pO_2 70 mmHg (9.33 kPa)
    pCO_2 51 mmHg (6.8 kPa)
    Base deficit-11
    which of the following statements apply:

    A   pure respiratory acidosis is present
    B   mixed respiratory and metabolic acidosis is present
    C   treatment with 35% O_2 is indicated
    D   pyloric stenosis and chronic bronchitis are present
    E   diabetic keto-acidosis is a likely explanation

39. **Lung compliance is**

    A   decreased by pulmonary congestion
    B   a measure of change in lung volume per unit change in
           airway pressure
    C   is decreased by emphysema
    D   is approximately half in a person with only one lung
    E   is determined using a peak flow meter

40. **In the fetal circulation**

    A   blood in the umbilical vein is 95% saturated with
           oxygen
    B   blood in the inferior vena cava is 80% saturated with oxygen
    C   blood going to the head has more oxygen than that
           flowing in the rest of the body
    D   about 55% of the cardiac output goes through the placenta
    E   the pressure in the aorta is higher than in the pulmonary
           artery

41. **The following are features of right ventricular failure:**

A   brown induration of the lung
B   elevation of the BMR
C   centrilobular changes in the liver
D   production of large volumes of dilute urine
E   depression of the ESR

42. **Which of the following is/are correct:**

A   vitamin D deficiency leads to osteomalacia in adults
B   in hypophosphatasia, the primary defect is renal
C   vitamin D-resistant rickets may be due to the inability
     to convert 25 hydroxy cholecalciferol to
     1,25 dihydroxycholecalciferol
D   hypervitaminosis D causes hypercalcaemia and generalised
     metastatic calcification
E   phytic acid in the gut is essential for calcium absorption

43. **Staphylococci are the usual causative organisms in the following conditions:**

A   erysipelas
B   scarlet fever
C   carbuncles
D   acute osteomyelitis in children
E   bullous impetigo of the newborn

44. **The following are examples of dystrophic calcification:**

A   the phleboliths which are commonly seen on pelvic X-rays
B   the calcified arteries seen in Monckeberg's sclerosis
C   the calcification of tooth enamel
D   the renal calcification seen in hyperparathyroidism
E   the calcification seen in fat necrosis

45. The following are examples of pure hypertrophy:

A   breast enlargement during pregnancy
B   enlargement of the left ventricular wall in systemic hypertension
C   benign senile enlargement of the prostrate gland
D   enlargement of the remaining kidney after nephrectomy
E   the increase in volume of the myometrium during pregnancy

46. Hypercalcuria

A   is a feature of parathyroid adenoma
B   may be seen in sarcoidosis
C   predisposes to renal stones
D   is a feature of immobilisation
E   is seen in renal tubular acidosis

47. The hepatitis-associated antigen (HB Ag)

A   may be positive in association with polyarteritis nodosa
B   causes infective hepatitis
C   can only be transmitted by inoculation
D   is present and positive in only one person in 1,000 giving blood
E   is always positive in chronic active hepatitis

48. Pulmonary oedema may complicate

A   diuretic therapy
B   rapid withdrawal of fluid or air from the pleural cavity
C   neurosurgery
D   radiotherapy to the chest
E   burns

49. Low output cardiac failure may be caused by

A   anaemia
B   thyrotoxicosis
C   advanced liver disease
D   Paget's disease
E   mitral stenosis

50. Ventilatory failure is usually characterised by

A   an elevation of plasma standard bicarbonate
B   a drop in arterial PO_2 in the presence of a normal PCO_2
C   hypercapnia
D   an elevation of blood pressure
E   papilloedema

51. Which of the following factors may determine the extent of ischaemia in arterial obstruction:

A   speed of onset
B   the pathological state of the collateral circulation
C   haemoglobin level
D   nature of the affected organ
E   an elevated blood urea

52. In Europeans, gall stones

A   consist mainly of calcium bilirubinate
B   made of cholesterol may be disolved in chemodeoxycholic acid
C   when caught in the cystic duct will cause profound obstructive jaundice
D   when blocking the common bile duct will give rise to bilirubinuria
E   when blocking the common bile duct will give rise to a raised serum acid phosphatase

53. Carcinoid tumour of the appendix is commonly associated with

   A no symptoms
   B raised 5 H1AA
   C raised blood pressure
   D flushing attacks
   E intussusception of the colon

54. The following serum enzymes may be elevated in liver disease:

   A 5'-nucleotidase
   B aspartate aminotronoferase
   C lactate dehydrogenase
   D pseudocholinesterase
   E alkaline phosphatase

55. The malabsorption syndrome

   A does not usually occur after removal of a short segment of jejunum or ileum
   B may result in bleeding tendencies
   C may reduce the quantity of fat in the faeces
   D may present with oedema
   E does not occur in tropical sprue and coeliac disease

56. A bleeding tendency may be caused by

   A drugs
   B pregnancy
   C massive blood transfusions
   D many severe infections
   E splenectomy

57. **The effects of chronic renal failure usually include**

    A polyuria
    B sodium retention
    C potassium depletion
    D alkalosis
    E parathyroid hyperplasia

58. **Osteoporosis is commonly seen in**

    A vitamin D deficiency states
    B scurvy
    C prolonged recumbency
    D chronic renal failure
    E hyperparathyroidism

59. **The following organisms are resistant to gastric acid:**

    A *diphtheriae*
    B *salmonellae*
    C *M. tuberculosis bovis*
    D poliovirus
    E *Diplococcus pneumonia*

60. **In mild hypothermia (32-37° C)**

    A blood pressure falls
    B shivering occurs
    C respiratory rate decreases
    D diuresis increases
    E recovery leaves irreversible tissue changes

End of Practice Exam

PRACTICE EXAM ANSWERS

1. A E

This region is badly named as its boundaries include the anal sphincter medially, the obturator internus fascia overlying the ischium laterally, with the roof superomedially formed by levator ani muscle and the floor being the anal skin. The two fossae communicate with each other posterior to the anus and so allow infections to spread rapidly in this region.

2. C D

The sensory supply of the face is mainly from branches of V, but the angle of the jaw and side of the cheek are innervated from the cervical plexus. Embryologically, the philtrum is derived from the nasofrontal process which is supplied by the ophthalmic division of V, however, during development, the maxillary branch of V takes over innervation of the upperlip. 'Motor' supply of skin means the sympathetics to arrectores pilorum which cause 'goose pimples' as well as sweating and vasoconstriction control of the skin. Buccinator is a 'muscle of facial expression', and is supplied by the facial nerve (VII), although it is an accessory muscle during eating.

3. A C

Most of inversion, the movement of turning the sole to face its opposite, is really a combination of supination and adduction of the forefoot. Eversion is a combination of pronation and abduction. Inversion is easier in plantarflexion, whereas eversion is very difficult without a degree of dorsiflexion. These movements occur at the subtalar joint and not through the midtarsal joints. The lateral longitudinal arch is maintained more especially by the ligaments and long tendons such as peroneus longus rather than the bony configuration which is an important factor in the maintainance of the medial longitudinal arch.

4. C D E

The diaphragm has its sole motor supply from the phrenic
nerves C3, 4, 5; it is the sensory supply of this muscle sheet
which is via both phrenic nerves and the lower six intercostal
nerves. Trapezius also has a sole motor supply from the
accessory nerve, but has proprioceptive sensory fibres from C3
and C4. Digastric is supplied by the trigeminal (V)-anterior
belly and the facial (VII)- posterior belly. Adductor magnus
has dual innervation from the sciatic and obturator nerves.
Biceps femoris is innervated from both the tibial and common
peroneal branches of the sciatic nerve to its long and short
heads respectively.

5. B E

The diaphragm is pierced by the oesophagus at the level of
T10; the inferior vena cava passes through the central tendon
of the diaphragm at T8. The intra-abdominal portion is very
short, rarely more than 1-2 cm in length. The oesphagus is all
lined by squamous epithelium.

6. A B E

The pancreas is an area of anastomosis between the coeliac
and superior mesenteric arteries. The left and right gastric
arteries, however, do not supply the pancreas, but go to the
stomach itself. The splenic artery supplies numerous small
branches to the body and tail. The head is supplied by the
superior pancreaticoduodenal branch of the gastroduodenal
artery and the inferior pancreaticoduodenal artery branch of
the superior mesenteric.

7. B C D

The left recurrent laryngeal nerve is a branch of the vagus, but
it hooks around the ductus arteriosum and aortic arch,
whereas the right recurrent nerve hooks around the subclavian
artery. The vagus is the most widely distributed cranial nerve,
and has a major motor and parasympathetic secretomotor
outflow. The preganglionic parasympathetic secretomotor
fibres to the parotid gland, however, are fibres from the
glosssopharyngeal nerve (1X) via its tympanic branch.

8. B D

The stellate ganglion is a combination of the T1 sympathetic ganglion with the inferior cervical ganglion (sympathetic) which occurs in approximately 50% of the population. It lies on the neck of the first rib often just posterior to the vertebral artery to which it sends some fibres. Damage to the cervical sympathetic chain causes a Horner's syndrome which consists of pupillary constriction, ptosis and lack of sweating and flushing of the face. A third cranial nerve lesion causes pupillary dilation. From the inferior cervical or stellate ganglion, the rami communicantes are to the C7 and C8 spinal nerves.

9. A B E

The ureter is developed from a mesonephric duct bud; the mesonephros being a mesodermal mass in the fetus. The ureter like the bladder, is lined by transitional epithelium. It is the ureter, however, that crosses the genitofemoral nerve as it lies on the anterior surface of the psoas major muscle. The ureter in turn is crossed anteriorly by testicular vessels which in turn themselves lie posterior to the branches of the inferior mesenteric vessels.

10. C

The tympanic membrane and mastoid antrum both develop from the first pharyngeal pouch. The palatine tonsils are second arch derivatives, and the superior parathyroid glands originate in the fourth pharyngeal pouch. The third pharyngeal pouch gives rise to the thymus and inferior parathyroid glands, thus explaining how occasionally ectopic parathyroid tissue may be found in a retrosternal position associated with the thymus gland.

11. A B C E

The medial rotation of the femur on the tibia is the 'screwing home' action which is said to 'lock' the joint. The ossification of the lower end of femur is used as a landmark in forensic medicine concerning stillbirths and perinatal death. Extension of the knee is via L3, L4 especially the femoral nerve, whereas flexion is via the hamstrings which are sciatic nerve innervated—L5, S1, etc.

12. E

The axillary artery is the continuation of the third part of the subclavian artery at the lateral border of the first rib, where it passes over the first digitation of serratus anterior muscle. The axillary artery is related to the cords of the brachial plexus, the trunks being found in the posterior triangle of the neck. From its third part arise the circumflex humeral and subscapular arteries. The second part of the axillary artery normally gives rise to the lateral thoracic and acromiothoracic arteries which supply the breast and shoulder regions respectively.

13. E

The suprascapular nerve is the only branch from the trunks (upper in fact). The long thoracic nerve to serratus anterior (C5, 6, 7) and nerve to subclavius (C5, 6) are both from the roots directly. The medial cutaneous nerve of the forearm is a branch of the medial cord and the thoracodorsal nerve to latissimus dorsi (C6, 7, 8) is from the posterior cord.

14. B C D

The larynx becomes the trachea at the lower border of the C6 vertebra at the level of the cricoid cartilage. It is at this same level that pharynx becomes oesphagus. The carina is classically found at the level of the manubriosternal joint (T4-T5). The trachea is not related to the oesphagus in the posterior mediastinum, but in the superior mediastinum.

15. B C D

At birth, (40 weeks), the ilium ischium and pubis are not fused and remain cartilaginous where they meet at the acetabulum. The blood from the placenta travels in the umbilical vein towards the liver and returns via the umbilical arteries to the placenta. These obliterated arteries become the medial umbilical ligaments in the adult.

16. B C D

The glossopharyngeal nerve is a mixed nerve as is the trigeminal, whose mandibular division is both motor to the 'muscles of mastication' and sensory to the peripheral part of the face and jaw. The cranial accessory nerve is a motor nerve that supplies muscles in the wall of the pharynx and larynx. It is accessory to the vagus (X) and the cranial part of the accessory arises from cells in the most caudal part of the nucleus ambiguus. The hypoglossal nerve (XII) supplies all the intrinsic and most of the extrinsic muscles of the tongue. The trochlear nerve (IV) only supplies the superior oblique muscle of the eye.

17. B D E

The obturator nerve arises from the ventral rami of L2, 3, 4, and sends branches to both knee and hip joints as well as the adductor group of muscles in general, including gracilis and obturator externus. Obturator internus has its own separate innervation via L5, S1, 2. This small nerve can sometimes be seen on dissections with the pudendal vessels as it hooks around the sacrospinous ligament on leaving the greater sciatic foramen.

18. B D

The skin derived from the maxillary processes is supplied by the maxillary branch of the trigeminal nerve (V). Branches of the facial nerve fan out like a goose's foot "pes anserinus" just anterior to the tragus. The most inferior of the five main facial branches is the cervical branch which may easily be damaged when operating on the submandibular glands. If damaged, this may result in a drooping of the lower lip. The facial nerve does carry sensory fibres including taste fibres from the anterior two-thirds of the tongue via the chorda tympani and pure sensory fibres from the external acoustic meatus and the mucous membrane of the supratonsillar fossae.

19. C D

The biceps femoris muscle is the superolateral border of this slim diamond-shaped region. The sural nerve originates from the popliteal fossa, but the saphenous nerve, a cutaneous branch of the femoral nerve, leaves the adductor canal and passes down the medial side of the front of the lower leg towards the medial malleolus. In the fossa, the tibial nerve is the most superficial of the structures in the neurovascular bundle, the popliteal artery lying deep and therefore hard to palpate even in the normal subject.

20. A C E

The male canal contains the contents of the spermatic cord which include the vas deferens, its artery as well as the testicular artery and vein. In the female, the round ligament of the uterus (gubernaculum ovarii) and accompanying lymphatics are transmitted along the canal. In both sexes, the ilioinguinal nerve is also found. The inferior epigastric vessels do not pass along the canal, but pass superiorly along the medial boundary of the deep inguinal ring.

21. A C D

The arteries and veins are large and therefore contribute relatively little to total peripheral resistance. The capillaries offer significant resistance, but have no muscle in their walls, and their diameter reflects primarily the diameter of the arterioles supplying them. It is therefore convenient to consider changes in arteriolar radius as the main determinant of total peripheral resistance. Peripheral resistance falls in exercise because of the much reduced resistance in the muscle bed.

22. B D E

The ECG is a record of the summation of potentials in cardiac tissue and so can give information about cardiac rhythm and conduction of impulses, but not of cardiac output and force of contraction.

23. C

Feedback systems are important components of biological control systems, both negative and positive feedback. The major characteristics of negative feedback systems are that they restore the regulated variable towards the operating point, either increasing it or decreasing it after initial displacement, but they cannot prevent the initial displacement.

24. A D E

Eccrine sweat glands are involved in thermoregulation. They secrete sweat which is 0.1-0.4% Na Cl - a proportion dependent on adrenocortical hormones. They are innervated by the sympathetic nervous system, but acetylcholine is the transmitter.

25. B D

Autoregulation of renal vascular resistance leads to a stabilised filtration pressure, which, however, is reduced when the mean arterial blood pressure falls below 90 mm Hg (12.0kPa). Creatinine clearance is used as a measure of glomerular filtration rate (GFR) and urea was at one time used. GFR is thus not influenced by plasma urea concentrations. GFR may be corrected for by variations in surface area. Filtration is opposed by the osmotic pressure exerted by the plasma proteins.

26. A B C D E

The region in the kidney which detects changes in perfusion pressure is the juxtamedullary body situated where the blood supply enters the glomerulus with the distal convoluted tubule nearby. It has been likened to a cuff around the afferent vessels to the glomerulus.

27. A B C D

Glycosuria may be seen after physical or mental shock as a result of excessive glycogenolysis. Sometimes, a tubular defect in the transport of glucose results in renal glycosuria. Tubular reabsorption of glucose is also prevented by severe renal disease. Glycosuria is seen in diabetes mellitus, not diabetes insipidus, a condition associated with a lack of vasopressin or a failure of the kidney to respond to the hormone.

Practice Exam Answers

28. A B E

Glucocorticoids as the name implies, act on carbohydrate metabolism, producing an elevated blood glucose by increasing glucose-6-phosphatase activity. They also increase protein catabolism, produce an increase in acid and pepsin and a fall in the size of lymph nodes. A fall in the number of circulating eosinophils results from the increased sequestration in spleen and lungs they bring about.

29. B D

Lactation is probably initiated by the removal of the effect of placental hormones and requires, in addition to prolactin, corticosteroids, thyroid hormones and growth hormone. Oxytocin stimulates milk ejection but does not initiate lactation. About 50% of nursing mothers do not ovulate until the child is weaned. Galactorrhoea and amenorrhoea characterize the Chiari Frommel syndrome.

30. A B C D E

Vitamin D occurs primarily in two forms: D_2 and D_3. It is important for calcium metabolism and deficiency results in osteomalacia in adults. A large dose of vitamin D may be found in the blood for 2-3 months, so an excess which causes hypercalcaemia and generalised metastatic calcification is difficult to reduce.

31. B E

The prostaglandins are 20 carbon unsaturated fatty acids containing a cyclopentane group. The evidence for a role in luteolysis in the human is inconclusive. Prostaglandins increase renin secretion.

32. A C

Water and sodium are absorbed in the colon and bicarbonate secreted. Vitamins are synthesized by bacteria in the colon, but probably vitamin K is the only one of any physiological significance.

33. B E

Bile salts and vitamin B₁₂ are absorbed in the lower small intestine. Fatty acids, calcium and iron are absorbed mainly from the upper small intestine.

34. A C E

Because the brain lies in the cranial cavity an increase in the volume of the intracranial blood leads to an increase in intracranial pressure; any change in the venous pressure produces a similar change in intracranial pressure. Hypoxia produces vasodilation and negative g an increase in arterial pressure, so both give an increase in intracranial pressure, whereas hypothermia produces vasoconstriction and so a fall in pressure.

35. D E

During the period of positive after-potential which lasts 35-40 msec, the membrane potential is more negative than at rest by 1-2 mV, so that the nerve becomes less excitable. A massive influx of sodium ions is responsible for the transient reversal of potential when the membrane potential becomes positive. The process underlying the hyperpolarisation is not well understood, but it is reduced by metabolic inhibitors.

36. A B C

The cerebral capillaries are relatively more permeable at birth and the blood brain barrier develops during the early years of life. Certain areas including the posterior pituitary lie outside the blood brain barrier. It can be broken down by irradiation, infection or tumours. The barrier is not readily crossed by penicillin, and catecholamines enter the brain in only minute amounts.

37. **A C D E**

The muscle spindle provides the central nervous system with information concerning muscle length; the Golgi tendon organ responds to changes in tension. It consists of thin fibres supplied by γ efferent fibres and possesses two types of sensory ending. The sensitivity can be altered by altering the length of the muscle spindle fibres. Muscle tone is usually due to reflex stimulation of skeletal muscle by muscle spindles in that particular muscle, resulting from an increased γ-efferent activity.

38. **B**

The negative base deficit and the high pCO_2 means that the reduced pH of 7.31 has metabolic and respiratory causes. This would be characteristic of a patient in shock, as for example recovering from surgery. Controlled oxygen therapy (21 or 24%) is indicated. Removal of the hypoxic drive would worsen the condition. Pyloric stenosis produces metabolic alkalosis due to acid loss. Diabetic keto-acidosis is associated with hyperventilation and hence a reduced pCO_2.

39. **A B D**

Lung compliance is a static measure of lung and chest recoil and is given as a change in lung volume per unit change in airways pressure. Since it is a static measure, it cannot be determined using a peak flow meter. It is decreased by pulmonary congestion and increased by emphysema. It is approximately half of normal in a person with one lung, as the lung volume is approximately half.

40. **C D**

Blood in the umbilical vein is 80% saturated with oxygen as compared with 98% saturation in adult arteries. Oxygen in the fetal inferior vena cava is about 67% as umbilical vein blood mixes with the portal systemic venous blood, which is only 26% saturated. The fetal head receives blood from the left ventricle which contains relatively high concentrations of oxygen. About 55% of the cardiac output goes to the placenta which serves so many functions for the fetus. The fetal lungs are collapsed so the pressure in the pulmonary artery is greater than in the aorta and most of the blood in the pulmonary artery passes through the ductus artenosus to the aorta.

41. B C E

The lungs show brown induration when there is increased pressure in the L atrium (chronic left ventricular failure and mitral stenosis). The basal metabolic rate is increased in right ventricular failure, and the ESR is depressed. The cause of these two changes is unknown. Right ventricular failure causes an increased venous pressure which in the liver causes centrilobular congestion. Right ventricular failure causes fluid retention and a reduced volume of urine of increased concentration is produced.

42. A C D

Vitamin D deficiency leads to rickets in children, osteomalacia in adults. Vitamin D itself does not act on bone: it must be converted to 1,25 dihydroxycholecalciferol, and an inability to perform this conversion causes vitamin D-resistant rickets. Excess vitamin D can cause excessive bone resorption and calcium absorption from the gut, leading to hypercalcaemia. Hypophosphatasia is a low serum alkaline phosphatatase. It is a congenital condition associated with abnormal bone formation. Phytic acid inhibits calcium absorption.

43. C D E

Erysipelas and scarlet fever are caused by streptococci. Staphylococci cause abcesses, boils, carbuncles, impetigo, acute osteomylelitis, pneumonia and septicaemia.

44. A B E

Calcification in phleboliths, Monckeberg's sclerosis and fat necrosis occurs in the presence of normal calcium homeostasis in abnormal tissues: dystrophic calcification. The calcification of tooth enamel is a developmental process in which calcium is deposited in the presence of normal calcium homeostasis in normal tissues. The renal calcification in hyperparathyroidism is deposition of calcium in normal tissues due to deranged calcium homeostasis: metastatic calcification.

45. B E

Breast enlargement in pregnancy is due to hyperplasia. It is believed that no further muscle cells are ever produced by the myometrium after birth. The prostate enlarges by hyperplasia. A remaining kidney shows increase in both number and size of its constituent cells. There is no increase in the number of glomeruli or tubules. The myometrium shows hypertrophy in pregnancy, individual fibres increasing their volume by a hundred-fold.

46. A B C D E

Parathyroid adenomas cause hypercalcaemia with increased calcium loss in the urine due to an increased glomerular load. This increased renal loss predisposes to calculus formation. Sarcoidosis may cause hypercalcaemia with a resultant hypercalcuria. Immobilisation leads to a net resorption of bone, causing increased loss of calcium through the urine. In renal tubular acidosis, there is hypercalcuria, which has been ascribed to increased calcium dissolution from bone by the metabolic acidosis.

47. A D

Some cases of polyarteritis nodosa are associated with circulating immune complexes containing HB Ag. HB Ag causes serum hepatitis, not infective hepatitis. Although the infection is usually passed by inoculation, it can also be spread by mouth. There is a low incidence of infected blood in the general population although this incidence becomes higher in professional donors and those who have received blood. HB Ag is only occasionally positive in chronic active hepatitis. There are probably several causes of the latter disease, but even if HB Ag is the cause, the antigen may disappear from the blood.

48. B C D E

Diuretics are commonly used to treat pulmonary oedema.
Rapid withdrawal of air or fluid can cause pulmonary oedema,
usually confined to the affected lobe or lung, by unknown
mechanisms. Neurosurgery or any cerebral damage can cause
pulmonary oedema, again by unknown mechanisms. High
doses of ionising radiation to the chest cause pulmonary
oedema. Pulmonary oedema may develop in burns, shock,
septicaemia etc., probably due to altered capillary permeability
following damage to the capillary-alveolar membrane.

49. E

Cardiac failure in which the heart cannot maintain a normal
output is seen in systemic hypertension, aortic and mitral valve
disease and in myocardial disease. In anaemia, thyrotoxicosis,
liver disease and Paget's disease, the heart may fail due to a
sustained call for an increased cardiac output.

50. C D

In ventilatory failure, the standard bicarbonate remains normal
(respiratory acidosis) until renal compensation occurs. A
reduced PO_2 with normal $P CO_2$ is seen in ventilation-
perfusion imbalance: in ventilatory failure PO_2 falls and $P CO_2$
rises. Hypercapnia is a raised arterial $P CO_2$, And causes a rise
in blood pressure. Papilloedema is an uncommon, though well
recognised, effect of prolonged, very severe hypercapnia.

51. A B C D

The effects of sudden obstruction are more severe than those
of a gradual occlusion, there being less time for the
development of collateral vessels. If the collateral circulation is
deficient, then ischaemia will be more severe. The state of
oxygenation is important because whatever blood is getting
through to the ischaemic parts will give better benefit if it
carries more oxygen. Organs vary in their sensitivity to
ischaemia.

52. B D

The commonest stone in Europeans is the cholesterol stone. These can be dissolved in chemodeoxycholic acid. Obstructive jaundice only occurs if the common bile duct or the hepatic duct are blocked. Obstructive jaundice is characterised by bilirubinuria. There is also a raised serum alkaline phosphatase.

53. A

Carcinoid tumours are found in between one in a hundred and one in a thousand of all surgically removed appendices. Although sometimes the tumour may initiate an acute appendicitis, they are generally incidental findings. The carcinoid syndrome is a very rare complication of appendiceal carcinoids.

54. A B C E

5'-nucleotidase, aspartate aminotransferase, lactate dehydrogenase and alkaline phosphatase are all enzymes involved in liver cell metabolism, and their release suggests liver cells are being disrupted. Pseudocholinesterase is manufactured by liver cells for export, and its level may therefore fall when liver cells are damaged.

55. A B D

A large proportion of small intestine needs to be excised before malabsorption occurs. Bleeding tendencies may result from vitamin K malabsorption. Defective fat absorption causes increased fat in the faeces (steatorrhoea). Deficient amino acid absorption may lead to hypoproteinaemia and oedema. Tropical sprue and coeliac disease cause the malabsorption syndrone.

56. A B C D

Many drugs cause a bleeding tendency, and in different ways, e.g. cancer treatment depresses bone marrow and causes thrombocytopenia; anticoagulents in overdose cause haemorrhage by interfering with clotting factors. Pregnancy can be complicated by disseminated intravascular coagulation (e.g. toxaemia, amniotic fluid embolism). Thrombocytopenia may be caused by massive blood transfusions. Severe infections may cause haemorrhage by endotoxaemia and disseminated intravascular coagulation or by endothelial damage etc.

57. A E

Early in chronic renal failure, there is a moderate polyuria and nocturia, due to reduced capacity to reabsorb water. Sodium retention is not a feature of chronic renal failure until terminally: rather there is sodium depletion, due primarily to inadequate sodium reabsorption in the face of the osmotic diuresis. Potassium is normally secreted by the distal tubules, and in chronic renal failure this becomes inadequate. Hydrogen ions likewise are insufficiently excreted, leading to a metabolic acidosis. There may be parathyroid hyperplasia, partly due to the fall in serum calcium induced by phosphate retention, partly because the active metabolite of vitamin D, metabolised in the kidney, is required for intestinal calcium absorption.

58. C

Osteoporosis is a condition of bone atrophy: both the mineral (apatite) and organic (osteoid) components are reduced. In vitamin D deficiency (osteomalacia in adults, scurvy in children) bone does not atrophy, but the osteoid formed fails to be mineralised adequately. Chronic renal failure has complex effects on bone which in general upset (generally reduce) bone mineral without reducing the bone matrix. In hyperparathyroidism there is increased bone resorption with increased bone turnover.

59. B C D

Although most types of organisms are destroyed by gastric acid, the gastrointestinal tract is the usual route of infection for poliovirus and *salmonellae. M. tuberculosis* is also resistant to gastric acid, and if ingested causes primary or secondary infection of the terminal ileum.

60. B D

The normal response of the body to hypothermia is shivering, which increases heat production. Blood pressure rises, and there is a diuresis. Mild hypothermia leaves no irreversible tissue damage: for example, hypothermia is used during open heart surgery.

ANOTHER PASTEST PUBLICATION

TO HELP YOU WITH YOUR PRIMARY FRCS STUDIES

PRIMARY FRCS PRACTICE EXAMS.
- 5 complete practice exams of multiple choice questions.
- All questions are different to those in the Pastest Revision book.
- Correct answers and teaching explanations for each question.
- Hints on examination technique.
- Suggested reference and reading list.

For your copy send the form below to:-
PASTEST SERVICE
304 GALLEY HILL,
HEMEL HEMPSTEAD, HERTS.
HP1 3LE ENGLAND.
TEL: 0442-52113 or 55550

Please send me .... copy(s) of Primary FRCS Practice Exams @ £7.95p.
+ 50p. p. and p. UK and £1. (overseas), or debit my Access/Barclaycard

No. ....

Name ....

Address ....

....

FRB